Medical Astrology

by

Heinrich Däath

Astrology Classics
Bel Air, MD

ASTROLOGY

THE word literally means a knowledge of the stars, a discourse concerning the stars, or the science of the stars. Aster, star; logos, reason.

Astrology is not only a science, it is a philosophy and to some a religion. It has many branches and may be studied under seven of these to advantage.

(1) ASTRO-METEOROLOGY, the study of the influence of the heavenly bodies upon weather changes, storms and earthquakes.

(2) MUNDANE ASTROLOGY, also called National, State, or Civic Astrology, which studies the influence of New Moons, Eclipses, Ingresses, Planetary Conjunctions and Comets upon the fate of nations, countries and peoples.

(3) HORARY ASTROLOGY, the answering of questions and the solving of doubts arising in the mind upon any subject from a study of a map of the heavens for the moment when the question is asked.

(4) GENETHLIACAL OR NATAL ASTROLOGY, the science of the influence of the heavenly bodies upon the individual man, based upon his horoscope of birth.

(5) MEDICAL ASTROLOGY, the relation of planetary influence to bodily health and disease.

(6) ESOTERIC ASTROLOGY, the more religious and philosophical side of the subject, generally studied now-a-days in the light of the law of Karma and the evolution of the soul through reincarnation.

(7) OCCULT ASTROLOGY deals with the higher mysteries and with the bearing of Astrology upon practical occultism.

Astrology is the science that investigates the action and reaction constantly going on between the celestial bodies and the rest of manifested nature, including man, and reveals the laws under which this takes place. Its antiquity is such as to place it among the very earliest records of human learning.. It was for long ages a secret science in the East, and in its final expression remains so to this day.

ALAN LEO'S ASTROLOGICAL MANUALS, IX.

Medical Astrology

BY

HEINRICH DÄATH

" All is through constellación
  Whereof that some man hath the wele,
  And some men have diseses fele."

Gower.

THIRD EDITION

LONDON;

L. N. FOWLER & Co.

7, IMPERIAL ARCADE, LUDGATE CIRCUS, E.C.

On the cover:
The Agnew Clinic, 1889, by Thomas Eakins

Heinrich Däath was born on September 19, 1872, at 3:28 am GMT,
in Peterborough, England. His date of death is unknown.
The first edition of this book was published in 1908, the second or third
followed in 1914, the details are murky.

In this edition the 1914 text has been slightly enlarged from the original.
No other changes have been made.

As of 2013, laws in America prohibit or severely restrict the practice of alternative
forms of medicine, hence this note warning readers of the possibility of legal conse-
quences if they attempt to use this book to do so. The publisher bears no responsibility
but wishes to point out that "religious-based medicine" may be an exception.

ISBN: 978 1 933303 50 5

Published, 2013, by
Astrology Classics

The publication division of
The Astrology Center of America
207 Victory Lane, Bel Air MD 21014

On the net at www.**AstroAmerica.com**

TABLE OF CONTENTS.

EXAMPLE HOROSCOPE, p. 78.

Printed photographically in Great Britain for the MUSTON COMPANY
4 BELL YARD, TEMPLE BAR, W.C. 2
by LOWE & BRYDONE, LONDON

INTRODUCTORY.

THE morbid disorganisation of process and function in the body, known as disease, provides a constant problem that must ever loom large on the mental horizon of mankind. Yet although disease is always more or less definitely associated with certain physiological departures from the normal, its real significance is rarely or never wholly understood. And still less is the fact appreciated that specific forms of pathological derangement co-exist with equally distinctive types of character and temperament.

It is only when an explanation is sought in the stars that the true state of affairs is revealed. Medical science, setting out originally with a knowledge of stellar rule and depending for the most part, in the first instance, on an understanding of stellar laws, has, with the progressive materialism of the ages, gradually ceased to take interest in the matter, until in our day even the very tradition seems to have been lost.[1] The ancient Egyptians, however, had their astro-medical science in Jatromathematics ; and in more recent times Paracelsus termed that branch of knowledge which deals with disorders of the human organism as produced by celestial agency, *medicina adepta*.

It may be admitted that much and perhaps valuable astrological lore has been lost during these past ages, so that at the present time what remains is but a mere fragment of the whole. Nevertheless, of late years redis-

---

[1] Practically the sole remaining relic is now the symbol ℞, originally ♃, an invocation to the planet *Jupiter*.

covery has gone on apace and methods are becoming more sure and dependable. Moreover, if it be desirable to know in advance—years, if necessary—the time when some disease will grow active, its true nature, and the probability of its proving fatal or the reverse, recourse to astrology becomes an imperative necessity.

The position taken by modern science in its hypotheses of the constitution of matter to-day is far more compatible with astrological practice than heretofore. A few years ago the speculations of the boldest thinker were called to a halt at the atom, but now even this line of demarcation is long overpassed and we are face to face with the fascinating features presented by the (apparently indefinite) further divisibility of the atom into yet more minute and component particles— the *ion, corpuscle, electron*.[1] These little bodies, which charge the atom with negative electricity, and are in some sense the animating intelligence of matter as the mind or soul is of sentient creatures, will in the future help us to a closer perception and realisation of stellar laws. Astrology, after all, is not such an occult subject as many suppose. It should be regarded as the higher physics and chemistry.[2] Its claims will have to be considered and its *quæsita* met along those lines ; and any day may see us in possession of the key of the law which until the present has been withheld.

---

[1] Indeed, there are not wanting those who contend for the probability of the atom being a complete solar system in miniature —or even a *cosmos*.

[2] See Mr. G. E. Sutcliffe's interesting series of articles on the "Foundations of Physical Astrology" in *Modern Astrology*, in which it is shown that the fundamental tenets of astrological tradition are deducible as mere corollaries of the latest developments of the electron theory.

The writer has already dealt in *Astro Physiology and Pathology* somewhat exhaustively with the theoretical aspects of the matter, and in this manual, therefore, he proposes to offer only a practical outline ; and, since there is not room for a full exhibition of evidence, if he frequently appears arbitrary and dogmatic it must be put down to that cause alone. The book is, of course, primarily intended for those who are already more or less acquainted with astrological procedure,[1] as an aid to the comprehension of a difficult and involved branch of their study.

---

[1] Those to whom the whole subject is new will find the elementary details they need in the Introductory Manual of the present series, entitled *What do we mean by Astrology ?*

THE SIGNS OF THE ZODIAC.

	NORTHERN	*opposite to*	SOUTHERN	
Spring	1. ♈ Aries (+ *c*. F.)	(A. *c*. +) Libra ♎ 7.		*Autumn*
	2. ♉ Taurus (− *f*. E.)	(W. *f*. −) Scorpio ♏ 8.		
	3. ♊ Gemini (+ *m*. A.)	(F. *m*. +) Sagittarius ♐ 9.		
Summer	4. ♋ Cancer (− *c*. W.)	(E. *c*. −) Capricorn ♑ 10.		*Winter*
	5. ♌ Leo (+ *f*. F.)	(A. *f*. +) Aquarius ♒ 11		
	6. ♍ Virgo (− *m*. E.)	(W. *m*. −) Pisces ♓ 12.		

F., Fiery   E., Earthy   A., Airy   W., Watery

c., cardinal   *f.*, fixed   *m.*, mutable

+ positive   − negative

1, 2, 3 = *Intellectual Trinity*   7, 8, 9 = *Reproductive Trinity*
4, 5, 6 = *Maternal Trinity*   10, 11, 12 = *Serving Trinity*

Parts of the Body ruled by the Signs.

♈ *Aries*	HEAD	♎ *Libra*	LOINS AND KIDNEYS
♉ *Taurus*	NECK AND THROAT	♏ *Scorpio*	GENERATIVE SYSTEM
♊ *Gemini*	ARMS AND LUNGS	♐ *Sagittarius*	THIGHS
♋ *Cancer*	STOMACH	♑ *Capricorn*	KNEES
♌ *Leo*	HEART	♒ *Aquarius*	LEGS AND ANKLES
♍ *Virgo*	BOWELS	♓ *Pisces*	FEET

Cardinal Signs	HEAD	*Fiery Signs*	VITALITY
Fixed ,,	TRUNK	*Earthy* ,,	BONES AND FLESH
Mutable ,,	LIMBS	*Airy* ,,	BREATH
		Watery ,,	BLOOD

CHAPTER I.

Basic Elements.

THE basis of all our investigations lies in the circle of the zodiac and the planetary bodies:

♈ Aries	♋ Cancer	♎ Libra	♑ Capricorn
♉ Taurus	♌ Leo	♏ Scorpio	♒ Aquarius
♊ Gemini	♍ Virgo	♐ Sagittarius	♓ Pisces

These are sub-divided into:

(*a*) Cardinal: ♈ ♋ ♎ ♑. Fixed: ♉ ♌ ♏ ♒. Common: ♊ ♍ ♐ ♓
(*b*) Fiery: ♈ ♌ ♐. Earthy: ♉ ♍ ♑. Airy: ♊ ♎ ♒. Watery: ♋ ♏ ♓

The planets are symbolised thus:

Sun	☉	Venus	♀	Saturn	♄
Moon	☽	Mars	♂	Uranus	♅
Mercury	☿	Jupiter	♃	Neptune	♆

Primarily there is an analogy, a sympathy, a communication, an adelphixis between each zodiacal division and some definite zone of the body. The location of these is broadly but closely defined. The child in the womb is an epitome of the zodiacal duodenary. At birth the impressions of the celestial divisions are made. Hereafter it comprises within the flesh all the attributes of such divisions, and becomes an exponent of them. This zodiac, the *macrocosmos*, is concentrated in the *microcosmos* of humanity. Through the knowledge that such con-association exists, astrology is able to relate the effects of the one in terms of the other, or *vice versa*; to deduce laws and make presumptions; although these latter need find no place in the scheme when so many well-proven facts are ready to hand.

I

The areas of the body mentioned are, in brief, circumscribed thus : ARIES, the head ; TAURUS, the neck and throat; GEMINI, the arms and lungs ; CANCER, the chest cavity and breasts; LEO, the heart and back; VIRGO, the abdomen and umbilical region ; LIBRA, the kidneys and lumbar region; SCORPIO, the genitals ; SAGITTARIUS, the hips and thighs ; CAPRICORN, the knees; AQUARIUS, the calves and ankles ; PISCES, the feet and toes.

It will be noticed that the rulership of these zones follows the sign-progression of the zodiac. If the joints of the body were sufficiently flexible to allow the feet to be bent round until they touched the head, the analogy would be perfect. Or, on the other hand, if we suppose the zodiac as something we might snip across at one of the divisions and flatten out, it would imitate its actual form in the human organism. The head in each case is the commencement of the series, and the feet the conclusion. In the Kalapurusha, or Grand Man of the Universe, these are Aries and Pisces, and, of course, they immediately follow one another because of the circular arrangement.

The planetary bodies travel through the signs of the zodiac, and by the changes and disturbances they there produce, institute sympathetic changes and disturbances in the human equivalent. Each planet, too, is intimately espoused with some division or divisions of our zodiac, arguing a natural affinity between them. Thus, THE SUN is in accord with Leo, THE MOON with Cancer, MERCURY with Gemini and Virgo, VENUS with Taurus and Libra, MARS with Aries and Scorpio, JUPITER with Sagittarius, SATURN with Capricorn, URANUS with Aquarius, and NEPTUNE with Pisces ; these being the respective *swakshetras* or sheaths of the planets named. But they also have specific attributes.

Those which concern us for the moment may be detailed in the following manner :

☉ Vital	☽ Nutritive	☿ Neural
♀ Lymphatic	♂ Inflammatory	♃ Plethoric
♄ Chronic	♅ Spasmodic	♆ Comatic

Athough in the foregoing we have little more than the alphabet of MEDICAL ASTROLOGY, it will appear at once how some words may be formed therefrom, and perhaps even a little phrase.

For if we postulate an example, say Mars in Aries, we may readily deduce this much of the person in whose horoscope it occurs : *Highly excitable temperament; over-activity of brain; liability to brain fever.* Or let us suppose Uranus in Cancer, then *cramp in stomach* would be a judgment requiring a few moments' decision. Cognisant of the presence of Mercury in Aries we may diagnose *facial neuralgia;* of Venus in Aquarius, *varicose veins.* And so on.

That diagnosis is not built upon a plan which promises to be so easy and straightforward must be admitted right here, and will be demonstrated in the ensuing pages, but this need deter no one from pursuing the subject in a methodical and impartial manner.

CHAPTER II.

Anatomical Sign-Rulership,

I. Aries. I.

THIS sign represents the head, and will always act and react upon that portion of the anatomy. It is a rough division only, inasmuch as the brain, skull and face are equally embraced in the rulership. It typifies energy, the thrusting forth of mental or bodily activity through actual excess of life force ; restlessness, changeability. Its nature is hot and dry, sterile and inflammatory.

The Principal Bones dominated by this sign are those of the cranium and face. The nasal bones, however, are under the subsidiary rule of Scorpio.

The Muscles include the frontales, occipitals, attolens and deprimens articularum, zygomaticus, temporalis, buccinator, etc.

The Arteries.—Temporal, and internal carotids.

Veins.—Cephalic.

Morbid Action shows in epilepsy, headaches, various kinds of eruptive maladies affecting the head and face, alopecia, phrenitis, vertigo, neuralgia, cerebral congestion, encephalitis.

II. Taurus. II.

This sign typifies support, connection, endurance. The portions of the anatomy comprised under its government are the neck, throat, ears and pharynx, including the eustachian tubes, uvula, tonsils, upper part of œsophagus, palate, thyroid gland, parotids and vocal cords. The Taurian zone commences behind at the termination of the occipital portion of the cranium, and in front under the lower maxillary. The cerebellum and base of brain are under Taurian rule.

The Principal Bones dominated by this sign are those of the cervical vertebræ.

Muscles.—Sternohyoid, mastoid, trapezius, sternomastoids, œsophagæus, stylopharingæus, splenius and conplexus, longus, scalenus, biventres, cervicis, spinales cervicis.

Arteries.—External carotids and basilar artery.

Veins.—Occipitals, jugulars, veins of thyroid gland.

Morbid Action shows in diphtheria, sore-throat, goitre, wens, quinsy, croup, glandular swellings in neck, bronchocele, apoplexy, suffocation, angina gangrena, scrofula, laryngitis, polypus, abscess, strangulation.

III. Gemini. III.

This sign represents flexibility, dispersal, sensation, subtility and communication. It thus comes to be associated with the hands, the nerves and the lungs (including the trachea and bronchi). Gemini people are subject to nervous types of disease in very great measure. The external rulership commences at the shoulders and embraces the whole of the arms and hands, from the clavicle to the phalanges of the fingers. It is probable that some sub-rule over these parts exists which at present is not very well understood. The oxygenation of the blood is a prominent function of the third sign.

Both the thymus gland and the capillaries are also associated with Gemini.

Principal Bones.—Clavicle, scapula, humerus, radius, ulna, carpal and metacarpal bones, upper ribs.

Muscles.—Deltoid, biceps, supinator radii, subclavians, triceps, serratus anticus minor, pectoralis, palmaris.

Arteries. — Subclavians, brachial, right and left bronchials, intercostals and radials, ulnars.

Veins.—Pulmonary, basilic, subclavians, azygos, veins of thymus and mediastinum.

Morbid Action.—Bronchitis, pulmonary consumption, nervous diseases, pneumonia, pleurisy, fractures of arms.

IV. CANCER. IV.

The influence of this sign is of a nurturing, fructifying character. It is moist in quality, receptive, transforming, concealing, and metamorphic, but with little real vitality. The stomach and the process of chymification are the chief organ and function of the fourth division of the zodiac. The peristaltic motion of the stomach is governed by Cancer, and the anti-peristaltic by the opposite sign, Capricorn. It was for this reason (although it may be presumed they did not know), the ancient astrologers laid it down as an axiom that medicine was not to be taken when the Moon occupied this latter section of the duodenary. Nausea and vomiting are very generally associated with Capricorn.

Cancer holds sway over the whole chest cavity in a general sense, the breasts, axillæ, epigastric region, lacteals, thoracic duct, pancreas, and to some extent over the womb.

Principal Bones.—Sternum, ensiform cartilage, part of ribs.

Muscles.—Diaphragm, intercostals.

Arteries.—Axillary, diaphragmatic, posterior mediastines and œsophagian arteries.

Veins. — Diaphragmatic, gastric, gastro-epiploic, mammary.

Morbid Action.—Digestive ailments, gastric catarrh, dropsy, coughs, cancer, cardialgia, eructations, dipsomania, cachexia, chlorosis.

V. Leo. V.

Leo represents the heart of the physical organism. It is significant of vital power, ardency, interchange and generation. *Sol et homo generant hominem,* for this is the solar sign, and equivalent to the fifth house of nativity, which latter is concerned with offspring. The spinal column with its marrow and nerves is also under the rule of this sign. The sphere of Leo is thus a vital, extensive and deep-seated one.

Principal Bones.—Dorsal vertebræ.

Muscles.—Longissimus and latissimus dorsi, transversalis, interspinalis.

Arteries. — Aorta, anterior and posterior coronary arteries.

Veins.—Vena cavæ, coronaries.

Morbid Action.—Heart disease of various forms, palpitation, syncope, fevers, spinal meningitis, locomotor ataxy, aneurism, angina pectoris.

VI. Virgo. VI.

This, the second of the common signs, is nervous and rather barren in quality. It is associated with the bowels, and chiefly with the duodenum, jejunum and ileum, for Virgo is concerned with chylification just as Cancer is with chymification. Absorption and assimilation, selection and utilisation are the Virgo functions.

The preparation and absorption of the chyle is often much interfered with in persons belonging to this sign, or having one of the luminaries afflicted therein. It is greatly affinitised with hygiene, diet and sanitation. Other parts of the body under this government are the mesentery, peritoneum, spleen and sympathetic nervous system.

Muscles.—Obliquus, transversalis of abdomen, rectus pyramidalis, diaphragm (with Cancer).

Arteries.—Gastric, superior and inferior mesenteries.

Veins.—Portal, hepatics, umbilical, intestinal.

Morbid Action.—Colic, dysentry, diarrhœa, enteric fever, cholera, affections of the intestinal digestion, enteralgia (*neuralgia of intestine*), peritonitis, constipation.

VII. LIBRA. VII.

This, the third cardinal sign, represents equipoise, distillation, sublimation and filtration. The parts governed are the lumbar region in general, and the kidneys in chief. The Greek word for rein or kidney (*nephros*) seems to have been derived from a Hebrew verb meaning *to shake out* or *spread abroad* as rain. The kidneys shake out or distil the urine from the papillæ into the renal pelvis. The old alchemists would represent a sublimed substance by appending the Libran symbol, so: ☿ ♎ *sublimed mercury*. The sign ♎ by itself implied *sublimare* to sublime.

Principal Bones.—Lumbar vertebræ.

Muscles.—Quadrati lumborum, sacrolumbares, etc.

Arteries.—Suprarenal, renal, lumbar.

Veins.—Renal, lumbar.

Morbid Action.—Nephritis, Bright's disease, neuralgia of kidneys, suppression of urine, spurious ischuria, etc.

VIII. Scorpio. VIII.

Scorpio represents procreation, readaptation, and is concerned in both the reproductive and destructive processes of life. It therefore exercises special dominion over the generative organs. The principal parts under the care of Scorpio are the pelvis of kidney, bladder, ureters, urethra, excretory vessels of testicle, Cowper's glands, prostate, the iliac regions or groins, the gall, rectum, sigmoid flexure (probably whole of colon), meso-colon and meso-rectum. Scorpio diseases frequently implicate the back, heart or throat. Castration (♏) affects the voice (♉). The parotid glands (♉) will often be affected synonymously with certain diseases of Scorpio, such as buboes. A chronic exanthematous sore-throat, diseased nasal fossæ, etc. (♉), commonly accompany syphilis (♏).

We must carefully distinguish between the parts ruled by Libra and those by Scorpio. An apparent Libran disorder may be actually due to Scorpionic influence. For instance, suppression of urine and retention of urine are different things: the former is a true Libran complaint, occurring when the kidneys for some reason or other do not secrete the urine; the latter is Scorpionic, the urine being duly secreted by the kidneys, but retained for some reason in the bladder. The author has found the disposition of rulership in the allied parts of Libra and Scorpio to be as in the diagrammatic representation given in Fig. 1, on p. 10.

This will show why gravel or stone in the kidney will be signified by Scorpio rather than Libra, since it is in the pelvis of kidney that the stone is formed, a part which belongs to Scorpio government.

Principal Bones.—Tuberosity of ischium, brim of pelvis, symphysis pubis.

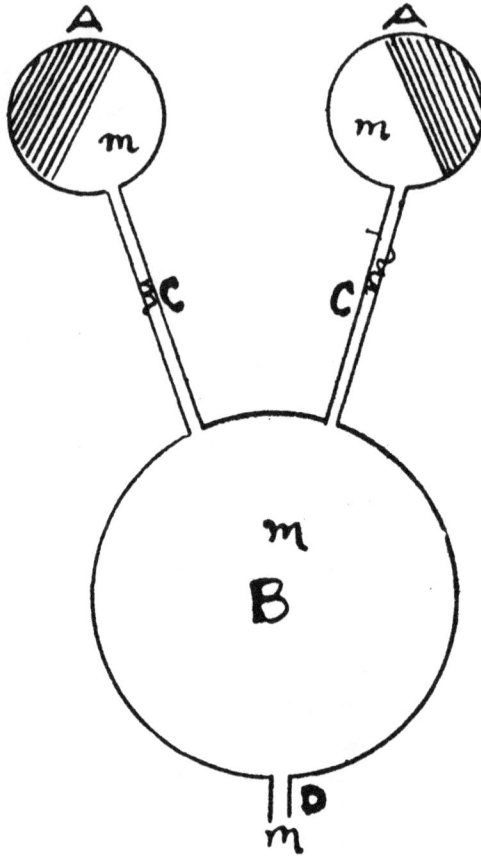

FIG. I.

A, A, the kidneys. The shaded portion represents the medullary and cortical substance. This is the part ruled by Libra.

The white section is the sinus or pelvis, dominated by Scorpio.

The remaining organs shown are *C, C*, the ureters, *B* the bladder, and *D* the urethra, all under Scorpio, too.

Muscles.—Cremasters, sphincter and levatores ani, erectores penis and clitoridis, sphincter of bladder.

Arteries.—Internal iliac.

Veins.—Spermatic, mesenteric, colic, hæmorrhoidal.

Morbid Action. — Gravel, stone, ruptures, fistulas, piles, priapism, scurvy, gonorrhœa, leucorrhœa, cata-menial disorders, vaginitis, uretritis, syphillis, injuries to spermatic cord, groin, etc.

IX. SAGITTARIUS. IX.

Sagittarius represents extension of sensatory faculties by means of transference from place to place. Gemini, in comparison, only reaches out with the hands, and has a relatively limited sphere of action and sensation. The ninth sign is closely identified with the locomotor muscles of the hips and thighs. Being one of the common signs it possesses some rule over the lungs and nerves. A remarkable feature of Sagittarius is special activity in the production of gun-shot wounds, and falls from, or injuries through, horses.

Principal Bones.—Ilium, femur, coccygeal and sacral bones.

Muscles. — Iliopsoas, iliacus, pectinæus, sartorius, rectus, quadriceps extensor, glutæus muscles (forming the buttocks).

Arteries.—External iliac, femoral, sacral.

Veins.—Vena sacra, iliacs.

Morbid Action.—Sciatica, enteric, rheumatism cox-algia, dislocations of hip-joint, gout.

X. CAPRICORN. X.

Capricorn signifies limitation, induration, nucleolation, servitude, and husbanding of resource. Its nature is cold, dry and barren. Just as Cancer governs in a general way internal mucous surfaces, so Capricorn does the outer and comparatively dry epidermis. The joints are also under the dominion of this sign, and particularly those of the knees.

Principal Bones.—Patella.

Muscles.—Patellar ligament, popliteus, etc.

Arteries.—Part ext. iliac, popliteal.

Veins.—Popliteal, ext. saphenous.

Morbid Action.—Skin diseases, articular rheumatism, gout, hysteria, dislocation of head of tibia, urticaria, impetigo, pruritus, eczema, leprosy, synovitis.

XI. AQUARIUS. XI.

The last of the fixed signs regulates the elimination from the body of carbonic acid gas and its products; has considerable influence over the blood and its circulation, especially where morbid changes are concerned, blood-poisoning, incomplete oxygenation, etc.; and governs the lower leg, calves and ankles.

Principal Bones.—Tibia and fibula, inner and outer ankles.

Muscles.—Tibialis anticus, peronæus tertius, 'tendo Achillis,' gastrocnemius, soleus.

Arteries.—Tibial.

Veins.—Internal saphenous.

Morbid Action.—Sprained and broken ankles, heart dropsy, anæmia, swollen ankles, cramp, heart weakness, spasmodic and nervous diseases, blood poisoning, caisson disease.

XII. PISCES. XII.

Pisces is a humid, lymphatic, plastic, torpid and cold-blooded sign, having a peculiar relaxing and softening action upon the tissues, and producing much phlegm and mucus. It affects the lungs, many consumptivès being born when the Sun occupies this sign. Those having the Moon posited in Pisces usually find colds and chills inclined to fly to the lungs. The feet and toes are under the government of this division of the zodiac. The matrix and secrets are also embraced, but more particularly where syphilitic contagion is involved.

Principal Bones.—Tarsus, metatarsus and phalanges.

Muscles.—Short extensor of toes, short flexor ditto, abductors of great and little toes, short flexor great toe, accessory flexors toes.

Arteries.—Internal and external plantars, tarsal and metatarsal.

Veins.—Of the feet.

Morbid Action. — Mucous discharges, gonorrhœa, gout, bunions, deformities of feet and toes, colds and colic taken through feet, dropsy, softening of glandular tissue, alcoholism, defluxion of humours.

CHAPTER III.

PLANETARY POWERS AND PRINCIPLES.

ALTHOUGH we have made another step forward it has not brought a solution of our difficulties. The list of disorders in the foregoing chapter is merely in the nature of an inferential zonal arrangement. Nevertheless it is a truthful representation; but because the inceptive agencies which create morbid disturbance are of various degrees of power and effect, we must look to other factors to aid us in the analysis. For it is quite evident that an inflammatory and congestive type of disease may attack one and the same organ at different times; that a nervous condition might be equally possible as a plethoric, and still our list would not assist the diagnosis. The requisite data are furnished by the planetary bodies, and as it is of the greatest importance rightly to understand exactly how they operate, and what they accomplish, it will be necessary to devote the next few pages to an interpretation of their influence from a point of view especially related to our present study.

First, let us consider the SUN, "the Leader, Chief and Governor of the other lights, the mind of the world, and the organising principle," as Cicero writes in his *Somnium Scipionis.* This represents the great vitalising force throughout nature.. It rules the fifth sign LEO, which is concerned with the birth of things. Its qualities are therefore vivifying and supporting. In the extreme form a hyperæmic diathesis will be indicated.

14

Hot, dry, constructive, muscular, life-giving, much depends upon its position and condition in the horoscope, and in great measure we look to this luminary to provide us with the structural, hereditary and vital physiological history. The character of its impressions on the organism partakes of the ardent, feverish, inflammatory and cardiac. Indeed, the heart is directly under the government of Leo and the Sun. Just what the latter is to the solar system, the heart is to the body. It is *cor coeli* and *sol corporis*. The less afflicted Sol may happen to be in a chart at birth, the greater the vitality, the more magnificent the recuperative powers, the larger certainty of warding off disease and attaining length of years. It is the *lebensgeist*, corresponds to the Hindu *Jiva*, to the *Monad*, to the theosophic *Prana*, and to the *Archæus* or *Spiritus Vitæ* of Paracelsus.

It may be objected that all this is merely symbolical, and that while most people would readily admit the life-giving powers of the Sun under the guise of heat and light, yet as a direct agency over the actual life no such rule could be conceded.

LET IT BE STATED HERE ONCE FOR ALL THAT WE ARE NOT DEALING WITH SYMBOLS BUT ACTIVITIES, ARE NOT INSTITUTING METAPHORICAL ALLUSIONS BUT COMMENTING UPON URGENT FORCES, QUITE CAPABLE OF PRACTICAL DEMONSTRATION, THE CLUES TO WHICH WILL APPEAR AS WE CONTINUE OUR INVESTIGATIONS.

The SUN then, who in Sanskrit is Dwadasatma, the twelve-souled one (alluding to the twelve signs of the zodiac), Grahapathi, Lord of the Planets, and Bharta Amara Joytisham, Lord of all the Devatas, or good forces, is the essential factor in our conscious life. Its energy is but poorly represented by electricity, because this at best is a reflection through Uranus. Sol is the soul of physical being, containing in itself every form of manifestation of phenomena ; the representative of unseen force, and the directing and motive centre of the universe. It is *satwa guna*, vital energy, *calidum innatum*, vital heat. Complex in the quality of its rays, it specialises through the circling planets by reflection and refraction. And just as the whole spectrum of colours is concealed in white, so the rays of the planets are combined in the solar orb. The attributes comprised are therefore observed to be the interchange and renewal of force, the conservation of matter, circulation. The Sun in the

> SOLAR SYSTEM : concerns itself with the *radiation of force* and *the indrawing to its sphere* of *worn-out residues.*
> SIMPLE ANIMAL OR VEGETABLE CELL : with the *nucleus.*
> HUMAN FRAME : with the *heart, blood-circulation, vitality.*
> WORLD OF HUMANITY : with *circulation of money ; commerce.*

Beyond this the greater luminary is connected with the eyes. Chaksu (*Eyes*) was a synonym for the Sun among the Sanskrit writers. With the Hindus it is *karma sakshi*, the great witness who sees all actions. Both luminaries in fact sway certain diseases and malformations of the "windows of the soul," but the Sun is chiefly concerned with the graver structural defects, and the Moon with the lachrymal apparatus and such defective powers of adaptation as myopia, presbyopia, etc.

The MOON is the medium of relationship, the conveyor and distributor, and because of its brisk passage through the circle of the zodiac it rapidly takes up magnetic force from the other bodies as aspects are formed and dissolved, and as quickly lets go, thus producing change, and acting as an expulsive, alterative and cleansing agency. It is the *mumia evestrum* of Paracelsus. The lunar person is ever a rover, restless, variable, mobile, inconstant. Our satellite, then, becomes chemically convertive, integrative, secreting, metamorphic and assimilative in action. It is the receiver and preparer, and is therefore intimately allied to the stomach, uterus and breasts, and so of peculiarly powerful import in a woman's nativity. As Leo and the Sun are identified with the masculine, electric, positive or active, so Cancer and the Moon are with the feminine, magnetic, negative or passive. The one is vital heat, the other radical moisture ; the one the sperm, the other the matrix of nature. Serous and mucous surfaces are dominated by Luna, too ; also the lymphatics and lacteals.

Taken in the abstract the luminaries together are ☉ Spirit and ☽ Matter. One is the reality—noumenal, essential, eternally existent ; the other illusion, *mâyâ*, transitory experience, organic decay. From them result two series of planetary expression : a solar and a lunar : the former always clamouring for deliverance from the latter, which implies bondage to matter, thraldom of flesh, fate.

The Moon then may figuratively be regarded as a sort of alembic in which the processes of fermentation and decomposition are carried on. Those substances under lunar sway are extremely liable to fermentation and putrefaction : cabbage, fungi, etc., for example ; these grow with astonishing celerity (mostly by night), have much consistency but little vitality or stamina, and ferment and putrefy with the utmost rapidity. They may be accounted the lymphatic temperament of the vegetable world.

Luna has a special rule over the stomach and alimentary canal, the brain substance, the breasts, lymphatic

B

and lacteal systems, and the lachrymal apparatus ; also
a general one over the fluids of the body.

MERCURY, the *spiritus* of Paracelsus, is somewhat of
a Protean artist, taking various forms according to the
manner in which it is aspected. This body is a con-
nector and mediator, a translator and reflector, a
distributor and co-ordinator. The specialised Mercurian
function is in connection with the nerves. Gemini,
whose lord Mercury is, indicates this trait. For since
this sign and its associated house hold sway in the
world over means of transit and communication, *i.e.*,
rail, road, telegraph, correspondence, etc., so in the
physical body these are represented by the ramifications
of nerve tissue. Insignificant as the body of the planet
appears, yet its influence is of the most important
character from a physiological standpoint. And although movement and muscular force are denoted by
Mars, the excitement is evidently due to nerve force.
On the motor nerves depends not only the nutrition of
muscle, but also the actual control. The intensified
form of muscular contraction termed spasm is directly
the result of the nervous system, and dominated by the
octave of Mercury—Uranus. Under Mercury we find
the nervous system, mental faculties, breath, hands and
tongue.

Together, the Moon and Mercury govern the brain
substance and function; and their affliction in any
scheme of nativity is a powerful argument of unbalanced
mentality, amounting to actual madness if the malefics
are dominant. It is perhaps one of the easiest conditions to detect in a horoscope, and one of the questions
most readily yielding a solution.

VENUS, the *adech* and Adam's Essence of Paracelsus,
is of a warm, moist and relaxing quality, soothing,

fertile, nutritive and nurturing. But its evil aspects and conassociations with other bodies have power to affect the organism adversely. It will produce general relaxation, loss of stimulus, the emission of vital fluids, etc. The planet holds dominion over the venous system, the kidneys, throat, and in women the ovaries. Its tendency, too, is in the direction of glandular swellings and malacostic action.

MARS, the "planete bataillous," the Hindu *Rudhira* (blood red), *Lohitanga* (ruddy complexioned), *Bhumi-putra* (son of the earth), comes next in order. He is "the red sphere terrible to the earth" (*Cicero*), the *Hor-Tos* (bruising planet) of the Egyptians, and the representative of animal strength and courage. Tension, heat, eruptive action are associated with this body. It is the proceleusmatic, augmenting and exciting agency, the great pathognomic symptom being inflammation. The house and sign occupied by Mars are always centres of energy, activity and augmentation, and thus become highly important in every respect. Mars represents focussed heat in contradistinction to distributed ($\odot$). His specific government is over the muscular tissues, the generative organs, the bile, nose and blood fibrin.

JUPITER, "that splendid star, salutary and fortunate to the human race," as Cicero terms it, is, like Venus, a supporting and aphetic agent. Its attributes are the conservation, elaboration and preservation of life, the ensurance of temperateness and fruitfulness. Some years ago a writer in the Journal of the Statistical Society demonstrated a connection between the fluctuations of the annual death-rate and the position of Jupiter in its orbit. This agrees well with the astrological significance of the planet. But when afflicting, this *stella errans* can exert a powerful influence by creating morbid changes in the blood, and causing accumulations either in the fluids themselves, or in the form of general plethora or localised swellings, adipose sarcoma, and under certain circumstances even the pancreatic, mammary, lardaceous and solanoid forms of cancer. To it are specially referable those disorders which are characterised by excess of sugar or albumen in the urine. The great centre of Jupiterian activity is the liver (storage of glycogen), but the arterial system is markedly dominated also, just as the venous is by Venus. Similarly the deposition of fat is regulated to a considerable extent by the Jovian star. Fat excites the liver to increased secretion. Frequently it acts through its oppositional sign Gemini, upon the lungs, as the latter will operate through Sagittarius : the excessive use, as a drug of mercury ($\math☿$) causing torpidity of the liver ($\math♃$). The formation of waste substances from used-up tissues, is exemplified by the production of urea, and uric acid, both of which are formed in the liver ; but the *deposition* thereof is due to Saturn.

SATURN, the *corpus limbus* of Paracelsus, is by nature dry, frigid and intropulsive. The action of this planet lies in the contraction, hardening, suppression, obstruction and atrophy of tissue and function. It is the negation of Mars. The tendency exhibited is to the retention, crystallisation and deposition of such sub- stances as would otherwise pass out of the body by the emunctories, etc. When this crystallisation and retention take place we have urinary sand, gravel, stone, among other things ; or in another manner we get the *tophi* or chalk stones of gout, thickening and deformity of local parts, atrophy of the muscles of affected limbs as in rheumatoid arthritis, thickening of the synovial membrane, etc. Because the principle of Saturn is limitation, its rule comprises the skin and bony framework, as these limit and define the corporature. The articulations, and especially the knees, are controlled, while the government also extends to. the auditory organs and the spleen. Saturn predisposes to chronic and deep-seated diseases. Maladies of the spinal cord are a frequent outcome when the planet much oppresses the solar orb.

Of URANUS and NEPTUNE less can be said, although various sidelights will be thrown upon their action in subsequent pages. They are responsible for the more obscure morbid manifestations, and such as are not amenable to strict classification.

The following tabulation will serve to give a slight general idea of planetary types of disease :

SUN.—Fevers, heart, spinal and dorsal troubles, bilious affections, eye disorders—choroiditis, ophthalmia, glaucoma keratitis, cataract, iritis, etc.—swoonings.

MOON.—Dropsy, chlorosis, œdema, vomiting, hydrocephalus, scrofula, tumours and abscesses, defects of eyesight—myopia, etc. (in Aries, conjunctivitis), feminine complaints, colds, catarrhs, mucous, serous and menstrual discharges and effusions, fluidic derangements, lunacy, stomachic affections, vertigo, epilepsy, periodic complaints.

MERCURY.—Nervous disorders, mental and respiratory complaints, impediments in speech, headaches, worry.

VENUS.—Neck and throat complaints, enlarged tonsils, cysts, relaxed throat, swellings, diphtheria, renal disorders, syphilis, maladies arising from free living, laxity of muscular tissue.

MARS.—Inflammation and acute fevers, operations, wounds, burns, nasal, muscular and genital disorders, hæmorrhage, fistula, rupture of blood vessels, infectious and contagious diseases in general.

JUPITER.—Disorders of blood, liver derangements, plethoric state of body or part, dental maladies, pleurisy, boils abscesses.

SATURN.—Obstinate and chronic complaints, rheumatism, gout, bronchitis, paralysis, deafness, hypochondria, cutaneous disorders, ague, palsy, colds, consumption, gangrene, mortification, atrophy, caries, spinal maladies.

URANUS.—Spasmodic disorders, ruptures, strictures, clonic spasm, cramp, shock, hiccough, subsultus.

NEPTUNE.—Obscure diseases having a psychic rather than a physical origin; but also coma, lethargy, cataphora, carus, catalepsy, poisoning obsession, somnambulism, ecstasy. Deaths and ill habits of body through the use of drugs—opium, morphia, etc. Stupor, typhomania, confusion of ideas, somnolency, hallucination, trance.

Briefly, the salient pathognomic signs attendant upon morbid planetary action (according as it is *plus* or *minus*) are, in the case of the

SUN.—Augmented vitality, hyperæmia.

MOON.—Chlorosis, profluvial effusions, œdema, diluted blood, transuding of fluids through walls of vessels, vomiting, infiltration of serum, defective red particles of blood.

MERCURY.—Reflex action, sympathetic irritation, neurasthenia, mental excitement, hurried respiration, restlessness, trembling, delirium.

VENUS.—Laxity of fibre, mechanical displacement, changes in the process of textural nutrition, cystic and hollow-tumour formation, escape of vital fluids, asthenic plethora.

MARS.—Inflammation, augmented sensibility and mobility, excitation, distension, expansion, determination of blood to part.

JUPITER.—Disordered circulation, changes in blood particles, plethoric distension, fatty degeneration, vascular fulness, leading to increased beating of carotid arteries, hæmorrhage, epistaxis, apoplexy, sugar in blood, sthenic plethora, etc.

SATURN.—Depression, diminished secretion, contraction of tissue, deposits, induration, thickening of cuticle, cell-walls, etc., diminished sensibility, lowered vitality.

URANUS.—Spasm, stricture, paroxysm, contortion, intussusception, rupture, perverted nutrition.

NEPTUNE.—Catalepsy, coma, analgesia.

CHAPTER IV.

BIODYNAMIC ACTION OF PLANETS.

THE biodynamic action of the several planets may in some measure be expressed diagrammatically. "When the Concealed of the Concealed wished to reveal Himself," says the Sohar, "He first made a single point; the Infinite was entirely known, and diffused no light beyond this luminous point, and violently broke through into vision." Let us suppose primordial matter, the Phœnician *moot*, to be represented by this dot or point, ultimately animated by the $\pi\nu\epsilon\nu\mu\alpha$ into the surrounding circle—the symbol we use for the Sun $\odot$. If we take this symbol to represent the sphere of each planetary force in turn we shall realise the following conceptions.

The solar action is expansive, expanding and circumferential. From the potential vigour concealed in the dot the force radiates concentrically in ever-widening circles of influence. We can exhibit this diagrammatically as in Fig. 2.

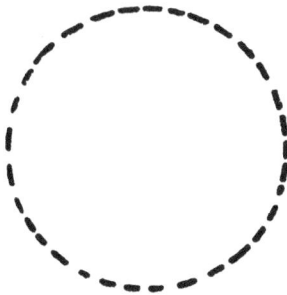

FIG. 2.

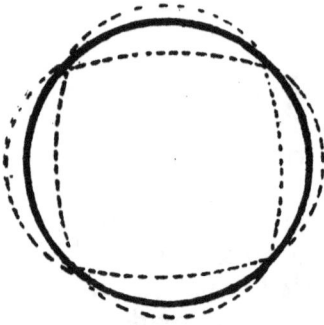

FIG. 3.

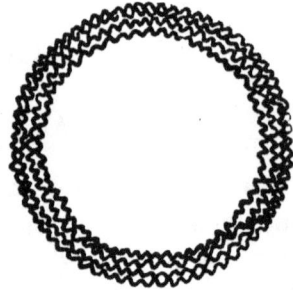

FIG 4.

It is expressive of life, infinity, continuity and enlargement of experience.

The lunar action is of the fluidic, ebb and flow order, mutational, periodic. It is the tide-swing as it exists throughout all nature, although for the most part only traceable among the fluids. Let us accord it graphic presentation as shown in Fig. 3.

Mercury is the tremolo, the vibrant, the unresting, the leading note or sub-tonic of the musical scale which demands that haven of rest, the tonic. It is nervous, quivering, excitable, subtle, in ceaseless motion as the ciliated disc of a rotifer. We may picture it as in Fig. 4.

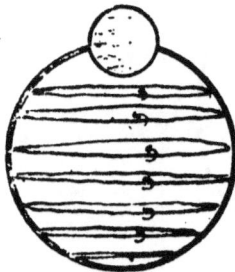

FIG. 5.

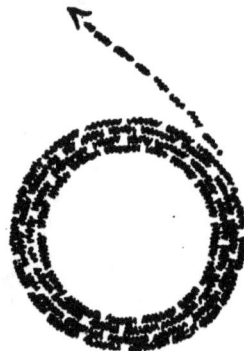

FIG. 8.

Venus affords us rotational or vortex-motion; and it is worth noting that Hæckel himself strongly insisted that this motion existed among the molecules of the egg. Then, too, it presents the phenomenon of gemmation as witnessed in many low forms of animal and vegetable life, where reproduction of the species is carried on by a process of budding from the side of a simple cell, the bud ultimately becoming detached and constituting in itself an organism complete in every respect as the parent. It will not seem strange then to record that Venus is specially indentified with the ovary and ovum. The sphere of the planet's influence extends to those disorders attended by cysts, glandular and other swellings at fixed points. Such non-malignant growths as acephalocysts are quite detached from the structures in which they occur, and have a power of reproduction by gemmation, the young being developed between the layers of the parent cyst. The Venusian action may be portrayed as in Fig. 5. This figure illustrates the progression of biodynamic vortices from one end of the cell to the other, ultimately issuing without as a separate gemma. After the energy comes the reaction. This is relaxation, and will be represented by the oval (also the typical egg form). Venus is a notorious factor in the relaxation of tissue.

The action of Mars is centrifugal (*Mars vicissim ad circumferentiam a centro protendit*), from a centre outwards; but although there is an affinity between it and the Sun, the martial force is not circumferential, not a steady process of concentric expansion such as may be exemplified by the widening rings which follow the act of throwing a stone into a pond, but a violent expulsion along the lines of the radii, as indicated in Fig. 6, p. 26.

It is rubefacient, bringing blood to the surface and so reddening and inflaming. As we have gathered, it is of

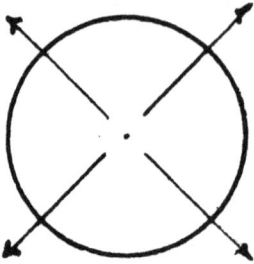

FIG. 6.

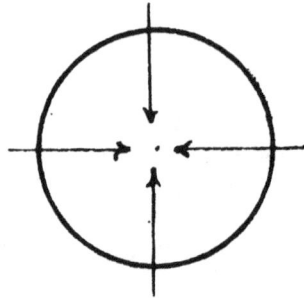

FIG 7.

an acute, positive, excessive, inflammatory, energetic, destructive and antagonistic quality, and is indeed one of the most potent forces we have to reckon with; while of course it will be understood as symptomatic of acute fevers and inflammatory complaints, violent shocks and injuries to the system, surgical operations and the like.

With Jupiter we shall couple in some degree Venus, for both are concerned with the nourishing, conserving and aphetic processes. To them belong the storing of various cell substances, the reservation, filtration, selection, transformation. The particular cell-reproductive form with Venus is that of gemmation. In Jupiter the process of cell-reproduction by division is exhibited. From the simple cell, by the continued interposition of septa and the progressive growth of each individual cell thus constructed, a gradual enlargement of the whole cœnobium takes place, until finally the rupture of the common integument results. In the human body Jupiter gives rise to conditions of plethora and adiposity.

Next in order comes Saturn. Here we have a force the diametric opposite of Mars: that is to say a centripetal one which continually draws from a circumference to a centre along lines of radii—"*virtute potius a circumferentia ad centrum omnia redigente.*" (See Fig. 7.)   The action is contracting, crystallising, binding, restricting, consolidating, driving the blood inwards and so producing colds, mortification, etc. What Mars allows Saturn negatives.   The one is sudden, the other tardy ; Mars intense, Saturn restrained. Together they are as acute and chronic, heat and cold. The two diagrams shown in Figs. 6 and 7 very well represent their several actions.

Besides being radio-active Uranus exhibits eccentric, tangential and spasmodic action.   As it is the octave expression of Mercury the vibrations will follow along similar lines, but the waves will neither be continuous nor rounded.   (Fig. 8, p. 24.)   Its province lies in the neuralgic, shock-producing, electric, spasmodic and explosive.

Neptune shows distinct amæboid and nebuloid motions, and while having affinity with Venus as its octave, it is more relaxing, elusive and protean.   It rapidly changes form, (not of course the planet itself), and may at times appear shapeless and amorphic.   Just as Venus is concerned with the process of cell-reproduction by gemmation, and Jupiter by simple division, so to Neptune belongs cell-development (independently of other cells) in a plastic fluid—the cytoblastema.

If we look back and compare the various characteristics, it will be observed that the planets can be related in groups :

VITAL ENERGY ☉ ♂		VITAL	☉
NATURAL AND		FLUIDIC, CLEANSING	☽
EXPULSIVE ☽	*or*	NERVE-TISSUE BUILDING	☿ ♅
MENTAL ☿ ♅	*again*	CELLULAR ,, ,,	☽ ♀ ♃ ♆
NUTRITIVE ♀ ♃ ♆		FIBROUS ,, ,,	♂
RETENTIVE ♄		CARTILAGINOUS ,,	♄

The Sun will represent the constructive energy, ardency

and life-force ; The Moon mutation, especially acting through the bodily fluids ; Mercury and Uranus the nervous system ; Venus, Jupiter and Neptune the transforming, conserving and storing functions ; Mars the muscular and destructive energy ; Saturn the retracting, retentive and scybalous agency.

CHAPTER V.

HOW THE PLANETS CRYSTALLISE IN ORGANIC AND INORGANIC LIFE.

THE Sun is not only the life-force of the universe it illuminates, but contains in itself all the powers and qualities specialised in the other planets. Each of these latter abstracts from the fountain-head certain properties, transmitting them in modified forms to our earth sphere, and, without doubt, to the remaining bodies of the solar system. *Solum namque cœlum est ignis: reliqua dicuntur ignita.*

With the method by which this is brought about we have nothing to do here. It must suffice that we are in possession of the ultimate facts resulting from this selection, forwarding and interchange of stellar currents. According to Sanskrit writers Graha Shakti or planetary energy is principally sent to the earth in the form of Vidyut Shakti or solar energy.

Given the indices of these nine centres (☉ ☽ ☿ ♀ ♂ ♃ ♄ ♅ ♆)—the individual and typal characters of their influence—it is really not a difficult matter for the philosophic mind to follow and trace them throughout organic and inorganic life. For we must remember that not only ourselves but the whole of animate and inanimate nature is acted upon. Many forms of matter and spirit are concerned, and reaction will assume appearances both varied and diverse, but the essential and intrinsic traits will never be effaced. Each planet will have to function *in materia crassa, in media,* and *in tenuissima,* and we must be prepared to recognise the gem by the sparkle of the facet.

Let us take Mars. The basic forms of the martial

action are centrifugal, inflammatory, intensive and poignant. In the human organism it will appear and reappear under such guises as muscular energy, mental combativeness, hot-headedness, anger, insistent will and desire, action, increase of red corpuscles, fevers, wounds, acute diseases, etc. Medicinally it is the tonic, aptly represented by the martially governed metal iron; temperamentally it is choleric; atmospherically heat and violent storms; mineralogically iron; in colouring it is red; professionally it is the soldier, surgeon, butcher, and worker with edged tools; geometrically the angle.

Or again, Saturn. This force crystallises mineralogically as lead, coal, rock; physiologically as bone, tendon, cartilage; temperamentally as melancholy, selfishness; pathognomically as depression, gloom, devitalisation; atmospherically as frost, snow; in colouring black; geometrically the cube.

Analyses more or less extended may be made in the following manner:

SUN (☉).

Qualities	Physiological	Physical	Pathological	Abstract
Hot	Heat-generative	Combustion	Feverish	Ardent
Vital	Heart	Gold	Syncope / Active / hæmorrhage	Passionate
Expansion	Circulation	Commerce	Dynamic / Superfluous nutriment / Plethora	Generous

Sign.—Leo ♌.
Mental.—Firmness, stability, will, perseverance.
Temperamental.—Bilious.
Typical Drugs.—Aurum, chamomilla, helianthus.
Typical Plants.—Euphrasia officinalis, Anagallis arvensis, Sanguisorba officinalis, Ligusticum Scoticum, Angelica sylvestris, Echium vulgare, Potentilla tormentilla, Hypericum androsæmum, Colchicum autumnale, Drosera rotundifolia,

Juniperus communis, Centaurea nigra, Chelidonium majus, Petasites vulgaris, Fraxinus excelsior, Sinapis nigra and alba, Calendula officinalis, Rosmarinus officinalis, Anthemis nobilis.

Therapeutic Properties.—Sudorific, cardiac, anticachectic.

Principle of.—Constructiveness.

Metals and Minerals.—Gold, carbuncle, hyacinth, chrysolite.

MOON (☽).

QUALITIES	PHYSIOLOGICAL	PHYSICAL	PATHOLOGICAL	ABSTRACT
Moist Secreting	Tears, muta- tion of fluids, etc.	Water Deluges Dilution	Fluidic secretions Dropsy	Emotional
Receptive	Womb (recep- tion of semen) Stomach	Seed- earth	Easily contract- ingdisease	Flaccid
Generating	Impregnation	Humus	Transuda- tion	Instinctive
Mutational	Inspiration Animal in- stincts Movement	Tides, Fer- mentation Decay	Critical epochs Dissolu- tion	Sequential
Relaxing	Sedentary	Moist- warmth	Atonicity	Apathy
Pacific	Inertia	Mother	Sedative and sleep- inducing	Night

Sign.—Cancer ♋.

Mental.—Timorous, imaginative.

Temperamental.—Lymphatic.

Typical Drugs.—Argentum, colocynth, pellitory, agaricus.

Typical Plants.—Many of the Salices, Brassicæ, Lemnæ, Saxifrages and Lactucas, Ophioglossum vulgatum, Stellaria media, Salvia verbenaca, Nasturtium officinale, Cardamine pratensis, Peplis portula, Utricularia vulgaris, Cheiranthus cheiri, Cucumis sativus, Anthemis pyrethrum, Portulaca oleraceæ, Cucurbito pepo, Mercurialis annua, Acanthus mollis, Convolvulus cœruleus, Geranium triste.

Therapeutic Properties.—Emetic, alterative, attenuant.

Principle of.—Change, harmony, receptivity.

Metals and minerals.—Silver, moonstone, aluminium, selenite, marcassite, emerald.

MERCURY (☿).

QUALITIES	PHYSIOLOGICAL	PHYSICAL	PATHOLOGICAL	ABSTRACT
Connective	Nerves	{ Motion { Volition }	{ Neurasthenic { Restlessness }	Sensa- tion
Subtle	{ Respiration { Breath }	Air	{ Bronchial Asthmatic Stertorous breathing	Intelli- gent Compre- hensive
Relative	Touch	Texture	{ Reflected ex- { citement	Irrita- bility

Signs.—Gemini ♊, Virgo ♍.
Temperamental.—Nervous.
Mental.—Subtle, intelligent, ingenious, witty, persuasive, restless.
Typical Drugs.—Mercury, petroselinum, avena, calomel, podophyllin.
Typical Plants.—Scabiosa succisa, Apium graveolens, Artemisia abrotanum, Petroselinum sativum, Pastinaca sativa, Parietaria officinalis, Satureia hortensis, Origanum vulgare, Cynoglossum officinale, Lavandula vera, Convallaria majalis, Glycerrhiza glabra and echinata, Anethum graveolens, Inula helenium, Fœniculum vulgare, Teucrium scorodonia, Corylus avellana, Marrubium vulgare, Daucus carota, Calamintha officinalis, Carum carui, Nephrodium filix mas.
Therapeutic Properties.—Nervine, alterative, cephalic.
Principle of.—Reason.
Metal.—Mercury.

VENUS (♀).

QUALITIES	PHYSIOLOGICAL	PHYSICAL	PATHOLOGICAL	ABSTRACT
Relaxing	Renal papillæ	{ Filtration { Exosmosis }	{ Remission { Laxity }	Ennui
Redundant	Res venereæ	{ Excessive atmospheric moisture	{ Swellings, cysts Erotic	Fecund

Signs.—Taurus ♉, Libra ♎.
Mental.—Artistic, convivial, amorous.

Temperamental.—Lymphatic.

Typical Drugs.—Cuprum, pulsatilla.

Typical Plants.—Bunium flexuosum, Achillea ptarmica, Verbena officinalis, Saponaria officinalis, Oxalis acetosella, Sonchus arvensis, Meum athamanticum, Dipsacus sylvestris, Sanicula Europæa, Prunella vulgaris, Senecio Jacobæa, Secale cereale, Primula veris, Ligustrum vulgare, Obione portulacoides, Plantago major, Nepeta cataria, Mentha pulegium, Galium cruciatum, Leonurus cardiaca, Sibthorpia Europæa, Althæa officinalis, Lithospermum arvense, Nepeta glechoma, Alnus glutinosa, Rubus fruticosus, Ajuga reptans, Arctium lappa, Prunus cerasus, Tussilago farfara, Bellis perennis, Eryngium maritimum, Matricaria Parthenium, Scrophularia nodosa and aquatica.

Therapeutic properties.—Demulcent, antinephritic, emetic diuretic.

Principle of.—Sex, love, desire.

Metal.—Copper.

MARS (♂).

QUALITIES	PHYSIOLOGICAL	PHYSICAL	PATHOLOGICAL	ABSTRACT
Enlarging	Muscular Sinewy	Action through the demands of sustenance, evolution, etc.	Hypertrophied Incrementitious	Excessive
Heating	Caloric	Trap-rocks Combustion	Eruptive Febrile Inflammatory Temperature increasing	Choleric Violent
Turbulent	Head	Fulmination Explosives, War Volcanic action	Exaltation Erethism Overbraced tonic fibres Hysterical	Frenzied Contentional
Energising	Hæmoglobin	Iron	Tonic	Forceful

Signs.—Aries ♈, Scorpio ♏.

Temperamental.—Choleric.

C

Mental. — Courageous, quarrelsome, rash, energetic, impetuous, antagonistic.

Typical Drugs.—Preparations of iron and steel, tonics, arsenic, cinchona, nux vomica, arnica, bryonia, sarsaparilla, sulphur, strychnine, cantharides.

Typical Plants.—Artemisia absinthium, Lapidum Iberis and latifolium, Ajuga Chamæpitys, Cochlearia armoracia, Rheum rhaponticum and undulatum, Juniperus sabina, Centaurea calcipitra, Cratægus oxyacantha, Gratiola officinalis, Humulus lupulus, Rubia tinctorum, Bryonia dioica*, Peucedanum Ostruthium, Arum maculatum, Urtica urens, dioica and pilulifera, Allium sativum, Carduus benedictus, Ranunculus aquatilis, Geranium Robertianum,† and columbinum, various species of Linum, Sisymbrium Sophia, Ulex Europæus, Gentiana lutea, Valeriana officinalis, Berberis vulgaris, Ocymum basilicum.

Therapeutic Properties.—Stimulant, tonic, rubefacient, escharotic, caustic, vesicant, aphrodisiac, resolvent.

Principle of.—Energy, anger, expansion, inflammation.

Metals and minerals.—Iron, sulphur, trap-rock, cinnabar.

JUPITER (♃).

QUALITIES	PHYSIOLOGICAL	PHYSICAL	PATHOLOGICAL	ABSTRACT
Supporting	Molecular nutrition *Vis conservatrix*	Hydro-car-bonates Sugar	Vascular fulness	Generosity
Sanguine	Blood en-richment	Fluviatile overflowing	Alteration red parti-cles blood	Buoyancy
Aggrega-tive	Cell-de-velopment	Thunder clouds	Apoplectic Sthenic plethora	Gluttony

* Externally the fresh root of B. dioica is particularly useful in cataplasms as a resolvent and discutient against hard and œdematous tumours, blood congestion from external injuries, ischiadic and other rheumatic pains, etc.

† "Our host at Carlisle told us that he used to be troubled with the stone, and the best remedy he ever had experienced to give him ease was the decoction of Geranium Robertianum."—*Ray's Remains*, published by Scott, 1760.

Sign.—Sagittarius ♐.
Mental.—Temperate, just.
Temperamental.—Sanguine.
Typical Drugs.—Stannum, eupatorium, mentha, ginseng, iridin.
Typical Plants.—Fumitoria officinalis, Salvia officinalis, Crithmum maritimum, Cochlearia officinalis and anglica, Hyssopus officinalis, Sempervivum tectorum, Lichen caninus and islandicus, Marchantia polymorpha, Acer campestre, Scolopendrium vulgare, Dianthus caryophyllus, Ficus carica, Melilotus officinalis, Cichorium endivia, Triticum repens, Lapsana communis, Taraxacum dens-leonis, Tanacetum vulgare, Potentilla reptans, Castanea vesca, Chærophyllum sativum, Borago officinalis, Vaccinium myrtillus, Betonica officinalis, Beta vulgaris, Agrimonia eupatoria, Asparagus officinalis, Smyrnium olusatrum, Saccharum officinarum, Asclepias vincetoxicum, Pulmonaria officinalis, Melissa officinalis, Geum urbanum.
Therapeutic Properties. — Alexipharmic, antispasmodic, analeptic, balsamic, anthelmintic, emollient.
Principle of.—Preservation.
Metal.—Tin.

SATURN (♄).

Qualities	Physiological	Physical	Pathological	Abstract
Cold	Low caloric	Ice	Impeded circulation, Congestion, Adynamic	Unsympathetic
Accumulative	Fæces, Scybalous matter	Dross of metals, Ash, Calces, Carbon, Soot, Cloaca	Uric acid deposits, Gout, Rheumatism, Stone, Gravel, Tubercle	Acquisitive
Petrifactive	Bones, Tendons, Ligaments, Teeth	Stones, Rocks, Petrifications, Mines	Ossification	Miserly

Qualities	Physiological	Physical	Pathological	Abstract
Depriva-tive	{ Malnutri-tion Starved condition }	{ Blights Solitudes Desert }	{ Atrophy Mortifica-tion }	Poverty

Sign.—Capricorn ♑.

Temperamental.—Nervous, melancholic.

Mental.—Antipathetic, gloomy, stubborn, laborious, reserved.

Typical Drugs.—Lead, aconite, belladonna, antimony, salicylate of soda, helleborus, hyoscyamus, conium, rhus toxicodendron, verbascum, Indian hemp, hydrocyanic acid.

Typical Plants.—Symphytum officinale, Taxus baccata, Polygonatum multiflorum, Isatis tinctoria, Asplenium ceterach, Tamarix anglica, Carduus heterophyllus, Prunus spinosa, Polypodium Dryopteris, Populus nigra, Cydonia vulgaris, Pyrus torminalis, Capsella bursa-pastoris, Illecebrum verticillatum, Mespilus germanica, Verbascum thapsus, Atropa belladonna, Hyoscyamus niger, Cannabis sativa, Helleborus niger, Equisetum vulgaris, Ilex aquifolium, Hedera helix, Centaurea nigra, Ægopodium podagraria, Conium maculatum, Lolium perenne, Ulmus campestris, Plantago psyllium, P. coronopus, Ornithopus perpusillus, Fagus sylvatica, Hordeum species, Amaranthus Blitum.

Therapeutic Properties. — Styptic, sedative, refrigerant, astringent, antiphlogistic, antipyretic, febrifuge.

Principle of.—Limitation, crystallisation, endurance.

Metals and minerals.—Lead, graphite, plumbago, lower strata.

URANUS (♅).

Qualities	Physiological	Physical	Pathological	Abstract
Vibrant	Aura	{ Radio-activity, Terrestrial magnetism Ideoelectric }	Telepathic	Intuitive

Sign.—Aquarius ♒.

Mental.—Eccentric, unconventional.

Temperamental.—Nervous.

Typical Drugs.—Ether, croton oil; also compressed air and gases.

Therapeutic Properties.—Electric, vibrational.

Principle of.—Intuition.

Metals and minerals—Uranium, pitch-blende, thorium, radium, polonium, actinium, uranite, chalcolite, lodestone, amber, shellac.

NEPTUNE (Ψ).

QUALITIES	PHYSIOLOGICAL	PHYSICAL	PATHOLOGICAL	ABSTRACT
Seclusive	{ Vermiform appendix (?) }	Odic force	Analgesia Atrophy of process thro' cessation of function, lack of cohesion of parts, dissipation of functional energy Clairvoyance	Semi-spiritual, occult Supra-material, Illaqueative

Sign.—Pisces ♓.

Temperamental.—Lymphatic.

Mental.—Psychic, inspirational, imaginative, romantic. (R. L. Stevenson was a typical Neptunian, that planet in his horoscope being conjoined with the Moon in Pisces.)

Typical Drugs.—Opiates, narcotics, papaver, etc.

Therapeutic Properties.—Analgesic, anodyne, suggestive, hypnotic, soporific.

Principle of.—Involution.

Metals and minerals.—Potassium, and such substances as meerschaum, ambergris, etc.

CHAPTER VI.

TONICITY, ATONICITY, AND PERVERSION.

A NORMAL horoscope would be the outcome of a due and proper balance between the planets—that is, such a balance as would not admit the preponderance of one over another. Each would exercise its activity to the detriment of none of the rest. But this is never the case. There is always some fighting going on. Each planetary body may be said to function in three different ways. It may through position and aspect be urged above the normal: this is its *tonic* side. It may be suppressed below: *atonic* action. Or it may suffer, in a sense, an unnatural change—*perversion*. In other words, in an individual scheme of nativity there may be too much of some particular planet's energy, an insufficiency, or a permutation.

Suppose, for instance, a man has a weak Mars. This will show as a want of spirit, lack of muscular power, lack of control over muscles, flaccidity, involuntary evacuations. If Mars is too much in evidence, fevers, agues, hæmorrhage ensue, inflammatory action is set up, varioloid disorders occur and a high temperature exists. If its nature is partly overlaid and intermixed with certain other bodies, but particularly Uranus, Saturn and Neptune, fistulas, morbid growths, fibrous degeneration, hæmorrhoids, priapisms, etc., are induced. Again, the tonic action of Venus will manifest on one side in venereal excess, the atonic in sterility: the perverted in moral folly. And similarly with the remaining bodies.

But apart from this, each planet is intrinsically tonic or atonic, electric or magnetic, positive or negative. The positive are Sun, Mars, Jupiter and Uranus. The negative, Moon, Venus, Saturn and Neptune. Mercury is interchangeable.

TONIC.	ATONIC.
☉ SUN ☉ Hyperæmic	☽ MOON ☽ Anæmic
♂ MARS ♂ Hypertrophied, acute, incrementitious, excessive, enlarging	♄ SATURN ♄ Atrophied, paralytic, cachectic, tabefactive, reducing
♃ JUPITER ♃ Sthenic plethora	♀ VENUS ♀ Asthenic plethora
♅ URANUS ♅ Perversion, stricture, disruption	♆ NEPTUNE ♆ Atrophy of process, dissipation

☿ MERCURY ☿
Receiver, reflector, amalgamator

Now an atonic or negative body may have its nature partially transmuted by configuration with a tonic or positive body. In a lesser degree a tonic body may have some of its positive force destroyed by the proximity of an atonic one, but cannot wholly become subservient to it. Each planet imparts a special type of disease to an organ, but becomes modified, changed or disguised by reception of cross aspects from other planets. From the combination of planet, sign, aspect and house we may infer structural and functional disorder.

CHAPER VII.

Zodiaco-Planetary Synopsis of Typical Diseases.

THIS synopsis is only an aid to diagnosis. The difficulty of framing invariable and universally applicable laws consists in the numberless combinations of planets and signs which are possible. Some disorders will be found repeated under two or more heads for reasons easily comprehended. But the list as it is here presented will afford clues; the working out of combinations, and the deduction of probable results must remain a matter of individual judgment. There are also proximate and ultimate causes and effects, which consideration opens up a wide field for speculation and investigation. In these astrology is at present defective; that is to say, we regard the results of disease more than the *causa prægumena*, the proximate seat rather than the efficient exciting factor. Diseases, in the main, ought to be distinguished by their causes, not their effects. For instance in such cases as stone in the bladder, caused by the deposition of uric acid, the condition of the blood ought to occupy first attention; similarly in diabetes: in this way we should have our observation drawn to Jupiter before Scorpio or Libra. Then too, it must be remembered that the graver diseases will be consequent upon the severer forms of planetary affliction. Not everyone whose Mars is located in Cancer will suffer gastritis; the intensity of the complaint will depend

40

upon the power of aspecting bodies, aspect configurations and other impressions of celestial influence.

SUN IN

ARIES.—Hyperæmic and organic headache, apoplexy, aphasia, cerebral meningitis, brain fever.

TAURUS.—Quinsy, diphtheria, nasal catarrh, polypus.

GEMINI.—Scurvy, bronchitis, nervous disorders, pleurisy, hyperæmia of lungs.

CANCER.—Dyspepsia, dropsy, chest disorders.

LEO.— Heart, back, and spinal complaints, acute fevers.

VIRGO.—Diarrhœa, complaints arising from mal-assimilation.

LIBRA.—Kidney diseases, skin eruptions.

SCORPIO.—Calculus, fistula, diseases of generative organs, nose and throat, appendicitis.

SAGITTARIUS.—Sciatica, paralysis, lung and nerve troubles, hyperæsthesia.

CAPRICORN.—Rheumatism, cutaneous disorders.

AQUARIUS.—Blood disorders, poor circulation, heart dropsy, asphyxia, poisoning from carbonic-acid gas, cardiac dilatation, (*slate-quarry miners*), caisson disease.

PISCES. — Urinary, uterine, pulmonary and nervous disorders.

MOON IN

ARIES.—Weak sight, eye strain, headache, migraine insomnia, catarrh, alopecia.

TAURUS.—Quinsy, swellings in throat, relaxed throat, aphthous ulcers, eye disorders.

GEMINI.—Œdema of lungs, catarrhal pneumonia, varicose aneurism.

CANCER.—Dropsical tendency, inclination rapidly to put on flesh, sickness, tympany, carcinoma.

LEO.—Swoonings, convulsions, heart affections.

VIRGO.—Looseness of bowels, abdominal swellings and tumours, typhous pneumonia, hydrothorax.

LIBRA.—Various kidney disorders.

SCORPIO.—Hydrocele, genito-urinary complaints, hernial aneurism.

SAGITTARIUS.—Gout, nerve disorders, ischiatic affections.

CAPRICORN.—Skin eruptions, synovial troubles.

AQUARIUS.—Varicose veins, ulcers, lower extemities, blood poisoning, eye affections.

PISCES.—Alcoholism, dropsy, relaxed tissues, colds, weak lungs, tabes.

MERCURY IN

ARIES.— Headaches proceeding from nervous strain, vertigo, brain disorder, astigmatism, neuralgia, phrenitic delirium.

TAURUS. — Hoarseness, croup, difficulty in swallowing through loss of nervous control, laryngismus.

GEMINI.—Gouty pains in head and arms, bronchitis, inter-costal neuralgia, asthma, pleurisy.

CANCER. — Indigestion, gas (*stomach*), stomach cramps, dipsomania, flatulence, neuroses of stomach.

LEO.—Convulsions, swoonings, pains in back, palpitation of heart, neuralgia of heart.

VIRGO.—Borborigmus, colic, diarrhœa, nervous debility, *ballonnèment.*

LIBRA.—Urinary obstructions, nephritic colic, neuralgia of kidneys.

SCORPIO.—Pains and disorders of generative organs, dys-menorrhœa, diseases of pudic nerves, neuralgia of neck of matrix and bladder.

SAGITTARIUS.—Pains in region of hips and thighs, sciatica, paralysis, nervousness.

CAPRICORN.—Rheumatism, gout, pruritus, psoriasis.

AQUARIUS.—Lameness in ankles, disordered circulation.

PISCES. — Cramp in feet, coldness of extremities, forgetfulness, phthisis, ailments proceeding from worry.

VENUS IN

ARIES.—Cold in head, lachrymal humours, musci volantes, eczema head and face, toxæmic headache.

TAURUS.—Swellings in neck, mumps, quinsy, relaxed throat,

salivation, bronchocele, exophthalmic goitre, thrush, ranula, retropharyngeal abscess, headache in amative tract.

GEMINI.—Whitlow, ganglion, papilloma.

CANCER.—Vomiting, dilatation of stomach, nausea, cyst and œdenoma of breasts.

LEO.—Heart affections, diseases of spinal marrow, aortic disease.

VIRGO.—Irregular bowel action, diarrhœa.

LIBRA.—Kidney disorders, high coloured urine, uræmia.

SCORPIO.—Venereal diseases, weakness of bladder, womb disorders, maladies connected with vaginal passage, ovaries, etc., leucorrhœa, prolapse, varicocele.

SAGITTARIUS.—Gout and tumours in hips and thighs.

CAPRICORN.—Nausea, bursitis (of knee), gout in knees (gonagra), skin diseases.

AQUARIUS.—Blood disorders, varicose veins, swellings in ankle.

PISCES.—Gout (podagra), bunions, chilblains, tenderness of feet, gonorrhœa.

MARS IN

ARIES.— Violent pains in head, ruptures of blood-vessels in brain, extreme restlessness, blows, cuts and wounds to head and face, insomnia, cerebral congestion, encephalitis, delirium, insensate acts, neuralgia, ringworm, S. Anthony's fire, small-pox, porrigo.

TAURUS.—Laryngitis, angina, amygdalitis, enlarged tonsils, diphtheria, epithelioma, pharyngitis, tonsilitis, rhinitis, acne rosacea, polypus, adenoids, epistaxis, muscular rheumatism in neck, parotitis.

GEMINI.—Disordered nervous system, cuts, fractures and wounds of arms, hands and collar-bone, bronchitis, bilious diarrhœa, pneumonia, inflammation of lungs, hæmoptysis, neuralgia, neuritis.

CANCER.—Dry cough, irritable stomach walls, hæmorrhage of stomach, gastritis, dipsomania, dyspepsia, schirrus of breasts or axillæ, bilious vomiting, hæmatemesis.

LEO.—Heart affections, palpitation, aneurism, hypertrophy

dilatatio cordis, angina, pericarditis, endocarditis, sunstroke, shingles (*herpes zoster*), muscular rheumatism in back.

VIRGO.—Diarrhœa, dysentery, worms, inflammation of bowels, enteritis, gastro-enteritis, peritonitis, cholera, ventral hernia, typhoid.

LIBRA.—Nephritis, pyelitis.

SCORPIO.—Hot urine, incontinence of urine, inguinal and scrotal hernia, hæmorrhoids, venereal ulcers, particularly in nose, throat and parts ruled by Scorpio, pains in bladder, stone and gravel of kidney and bladder, immoderate catamenial discharge (*menorrhagia*), ovaritis, scarlatina, diabetes, neuralgia of neck of womb, vaginitis, hypertrophy of prostate, uretritis, perityphlitis (*appendicitis*).

SAGITTARIUS.—Sciatica, ulcers of hips and thighs, enteric fever, pelvic operations.

CAPRICORN.—Flying · gout, rheumatic fever, contusions, smallpox, and other varioloid diseases, urticaria, pruritus, anthrax, psoriasis, scabies.

AQUARIUS.—Overheated blood, intermittent fever, erysipelas of extremities, blood poisoning.

PISCES.—Bunions, corns, pectoral affections; sweating of lower extremities,—bromidrosis, hyperidrosis, dysidrosis, etc.; diseases arising from exessive drinking, balanitis.

JUPITER IN

ARIES.—Determination of blood to head, congestion of brain, giddiness.

TAURUS.—Quinsy, gout, plethora from high living, apoplexy, coryza, epistaxis.

GEMINI. — Pleurisy, blood and lung disorders, fatty transformation of liver, apoplexy of lungs.

CANCER.—Dropsy, digestive disorders, overloaded stomach, dilatation of stomach.

LEO.—Fevers, apoplexy, fatty degeneration of heart, palpitation.

VIRGO.—Consumptive tendency, liver affections, intestinal maladies, abscess of liver, jaundice, fatty degeneration of liver.

LIBRA.—Changes in blood circulation, obstructions, pleurisy, tumours in kidney.

SCORPIO.—Venereal disorders, piles, urinal and seminal complaints, dropsy, strangury, fistula, urethral abscess, over secretion of urates.

SAGITTARIUS.—Pains and swellings in hips and thighs, gout, rheumatism.

CAPRICORN.—Eczema, and various other forms of cutaneous disorder.

AQUARIUS.—Lumbago, blood-poisoning, swollen ankles, heart dropsy.

PISCES.—Hydrothorax, hydatid cysts, liver and lung complications.

SATURN IN

ARIES.—Catarrh, deafness, toothache, colds and chills, cerebral anæmia, apathy, paralysis, rheumatic headache, cerebral syncope.

TAURUS.—Laryngeal consumption, scurvy, phlegm in throat, coryza, loss of voice, suffocation, angina, gangrena, putrid gums, diphtheria.

GEMINI.—Rheumatism of arms, hands and shoulders, consumption of lungs, black jaundice, dislocation of arm and shoulder, chronic bronchitis, nervous trembling, fibrosis of lungs, dyspnœa.

CANCER.—Asthma, consumption, bruises in breast, ague, loss of appetite, dyspepsia, nausea, chronic gastritis, anæmia, cancer of breasts and axillæ, eructations, chlorosis, dipsomania.

LEO.—Atrophy and weak muscular action of heart, weak back, malformed spine, syncope, jaundice, locomotor ataxy, gout in heart.

VIRGO.—Abdominal phthisis, costiveness, griping, derangements of intestinal digestion, mal-nutrition, sluggish liver.

LIBRA.—Bright's disease, corrupted blood, renal colic, sterility, suppression of urine.

SCORPIO.—Strangury, retention of urine, gout, fistula, palsy, piles, gravel, stone, suppression of catamenia, caries of cartilage of nose.

SAGITTARIUS.—Gout, sciatica, hip-joint disease, dislocation of hip-joint.

CAPRICORN.—Rheumatism (chiefly articular), skin diseases, knee injuries.

AQUARIUS.—Cramp, anæmia, weak and sprained ankles, club-foot from contraction of the *tendo Achillis*, asthenia, spinal curvature, caries of spine, compression and sclerosis of spinal cord, arterial sclerosis.

PISCES.—Scrofula, ulcers of feet, gout, consumption, rachitis.

URANUS

is responsible for sudden attacks of disease—cramps, spasms, ruptures, explosions, electric and other shocks, exaggerated action. When in ARIES or the first house it brings acute neuralgic, darting and shooting pains in the head; in GEMINI spasmodic asthma; in CANCER cramp of stomach; in LEO suspension of heart's action; in SCORPIO spasm of the bladder; and so with other signs.

NEPTUNE

has dominion over certain vague and obscure diseases, mostly having a psychic rather than a physical origin as explained before. When afflicting it will induce the habit of taking drugs, such as narcotics, hypnotics, opiates, etc. It is also symptomatic of poisoning.

CHAPTER VIII.

The Sixth and Eighth Houses.

THE sixth house of the scheme has always been held to govern disease in a broad sense, and the eighth the manner of death. This is quite true. But they are only worth considering in that light when planetarily tenanted. To attempt diagnosis by taking the lords of these houses is futile. Wilson writes: "The cause why the ascendant operates upon the human constitution is unknown, but experience proves it has some effect. It does not so clearly appear that the west angle has any such influence, and still less that the sixth house can be the place from whence we can judge of diseases."

To a certain extent each of the four cadent houses of the horoscope is indentified with disease, those portions of the figure signifying a falling away from a fixed or normal point. The common signs, which are equivalent to these divisions, are constitutionally among the weakest of the zodiac. But we shall ignore the third and ninth because the interpretation of diseases belonging to these departments is outside the scope of a manual such as the present.

The house chiefly regarded is the sixth, and the sign Virgo. This brings home one great fact—the power of the mind over the body, and *vice versa*. For the mental ruler, Mercury, is proprietor of this sign. "The diseases of the body act through the vital principle upon the mind, and on the other hand, the diseases of the mind act through the same medium upon the body. These are the only instances we are cognisant of in which

47

matter and spirit meet and act upon each other; in all other cases, so far as we know, matter acts only upon matter, and spirit upon spirit."[*]

When the luminaries occupy this part of the geniture, the vitality and stamina are reduced, chronic ill-health and poor recuperative powers coincide. Of course, should there be malefic rays thrown to the bodies named the evil is so much the more intensified. In many cases incurable disease is signified, or structural defect. And although congenital defects must depend upon an epoch prior to the actual birth, or upon some arrest of fœtal development, yet certain agreements exist between that which is born and the stars at the time. The indications are not always satisfactory, but it may be mentioned that the sixth and twelfth houses are often strongly in evidence, by reason of one or both lights being there conjoined with other planets. In deformities of body, such as hunchbacks, dwarfs, etc., especially where attended by undeveloped or retarded mental powers, the following positions will frequently be observed: (1) Taurus, Scorpio or Capricorn on ascendant; (2) luminaries in sixth or twelfth; (3) close association of the malefics, Mars, Saturn, and Uranus, especially by conjunction or opposition and in fixed signs; (4) their bodies or rays in or directed upon fifth, sixth or twelfth houses or cusps; (5) ditto to ascending degree; (6) many planets in Virgo and the sixth or twelfth. A few examples may be adduced.

Male : 9h. p.m., August 11th, 1874, Lat. 53° N. Long. 12m. W.—Mentally deficient; Pott's curvature of spine; cyanosis (arising from the partition between right and left sides of heart being incomplete); distorted features;

---

* *Essays on Medicine.*—Dr. Sharp.

almost a Cyclops. Here we have no less than seven bodies in fixed signs ; the luminaries in sixth heavily pressed by the rays from Mars, Saturn, Uranus, Venus and Jupiter. Mercury is injured by the proximity of Mars and the par. dec. with Saturn. Two malefics are conjoined in the fifth and opposed by a third, Saturn. Leo and Aquarius, the heart and spinal signs, are prominent and account for the cyanosis and spinal curvature.

Female : August 27th, 1889, 9h. p.m., Lat. 50°44 N., Long. 1°50'W.—Dwarf, hunchback, no hair or teeth, cannot talk or be taught anything, has little or no memory. Large mouth, coarse features, very animal-like. Several brothers and sisters, all normal. In this case Taurus is on the ascendant. Sun, Moon, Mercury and Uranus occupy the sixth, the first three being in Virgo. Mars and Saturn are conjoined in the fifth.

Female : October 19th, 1875, 6h. p.m., Lat. and Long. as before.—A dwarf about four feet in height, not hunchback, but her mind is that of a child of seven or eight years. Has had an illegitimate child which is normal in size. Taurus again rises. The Sun, Mercury, Venus and Jupiter are in sixth. Uranus is in the fifth opposed by Saturn, both bodies throwing quartiles to Mercury. Five planets are stationed in fixed signs.

Female : September 4th, 1880, 7h. 30m. p.m., Lat. 51°28' N., Long. 0°18' W. — Idiot from birth, the posterior portion of the brain never having been developed. No fewer than six bodies, including the luminaries, are in the twelfth house of this scheme, and all occupy the sign Virgo.

These figures will repay study and comparison. A whole series of strikingly similar ones might be given here, but the subjects of teratology, achondroplasia, etc., are entirely subsidiary ones in our present scheme. The

D

foregoing instances are introduced merely to illustrate one phase of sixth house influence. Such associations, however, as Mars conjunction or opposition Saturn, Saturn opposition Uranus, etc., in whatever part of the scheme, have a tendency to produce deformity, either congenital or acquired.

The twelfth house should be particularly noted for those diseases which demand isolation, or hospital or asylum detention. Planets in the eighth will usually point out the character of the death. Mars and Uranus will indicate sudden and violent death. Saturn lingering, wasting, suffocation, drowning, etc. But much will depend upon the sign occupied, as we have learnt previously.

CHAPTER IX.

THE TRIPLICITIES AND QUADRUPLICITIES.

THE zodiac splits up naturally into four tripartite
divisions which are akin in quality or constitution, *viz.*,
a *Fiery* trigon composed of Aries, Leo and Sagittarius;
an *Earthy* trigon embracing Taurus, Virgo and Capricorn; an *Airy* trigon, Gemini, Libra and Aquarius; and
a *Watery*, Cancer, Scorpio and Pisces. They have been
loosely termed elemental, but this is not correct: earth,
air, and water being of course compound substances.
Together we may relate and consider them somewhat as
follows :

FIRE.	Individual.	The spiritual aspirations.	
EARTH.	Physical.	Temporal.	Propagative.
AIR.	Relative.	Connective.	
WATER.	Mutational.	Terminal.	Translative.

Fiery Signs are connected with the vital heat and
spirit.

Earthy Signs with the osseous structure, the salts,
earths, minerals, concretions, etc., of the system.

Airy Signs with the gases, intercellular spaces, air-
cells, arteries, veins and capillaries.

Watery Signs with the fluids: (♋) milk, digestive
juices, ferments, such as gastric juice, ptyalin, pancreatic diastase, saliva; medullary juices, chyme,
albumen, etc.; (♏) excrementitious fluids—urine,
sweat, menses; (♓) mucus, pleural, peritoneal and
synovial serums, intestinal mucus, etc.

These are general considerations; but it must be understood that the particular character of a fluid will depend upon the planetary government.   Thus, although the Moon dominates all fluids, yet its real dominion is over the neutral solution, the bland and basic humour that constitutes a medium through which certain substances can act and react, and by which they can be transported to various parts of the body, dissolved, resolved and expulsed if needs be.   For instance, there is milk.   Here we have one of the highest forms of nutriment.   First there is the watery basis (☽), then the fatty constituents (♃), the caseine and extractive matters (☉), and lastly the salts (♄).   The futility of placing a compound fluid like this under purely lunar rule is apparent.   But when we do so we realise that the constitutional fluidic quality is the point of view from which we regard it, and not its specialised form as an agent or reagent.

The four celestial trigons crystallise in humanity also as the four temperaments.   The SANGUINE temperament is represented by the airy trigon and the planet Jupiter; the CHOLERIC or bilious by the fiery, and the planets Sun and Mars; the NERVOUS by the earthy, and the planets Mercury, Uranus and Saturn; and the LYMPHATIC by the aqueous, and the planets Moon, Venus and Neptune.   And every physician knows the type of disease likely to eventuate in each class, and also has some small ability to recognise the physical types of form, the physiological habit, and the mental capacity.   One cannot easily mistake the restless, neurasthenic, hurried, agitated and alert manner of the *nervous* temperament, its disposition to nervous disorders, etc.; nor the excited, rash, feverish nature of the *choleric*, with its bilious and inflammatory affections; nor the pallid, anæmic, languid, weak-pulsed, lethargic *pituitary*, with its tendency to dropsy, its deficiency of red corpuscles in the blood, its want of vascular action, tone, and the inherent disposition to serous diseases; nor finally, the *sanguine* with its active circulation, jovial nature, plump body, fine complexion, cheerful anticipation, and its hæmorrhagic diathesis.

But an explanation can only be obtained from a study of the trigons as previously outlined. The temperament is defined at the birth, and with it all that it implies, not only physiologically but in every department of life. For instance, from a vocational standpoint the temperaments will fall into broad divisions such as below: *Sanguine.*—Active, industrial. *Bilious.*—Active, political, military. *Nervous.*—Artistic, imaginative, studious. *Lymphatic.*—Scientific, contemplative, emotional, plastic.

The sanguine and bilious act, the nervous and lymphatic think and feel.

We have yet to make one final division of the duodenary, by which we obtain the series of three quadrates usually denominated CARDINAL, or moveable (♈ ♋ ♎ ♑); FIXED or stable (♉ ♌ ♏ ♒); and MUTABLE, or common (♊ ♍ ♐ ♓).*

The Hindu Trinity corresponds to this distribution. Aries is the *Brahma*, mover, evolver, creator, head; then succeeds Taurus, *Vishnu*, the protector, something fixed and made permanent; then Gemini, *Iswara*, the destroyer, that is, change from a previous state of fixedness. We arrive next at Cancer, the second cardinal sign and the commencement of a new trinity. It thus appears that all the *Chara*, moving or Cardinal signs are Brahmic; the Fixed ones (*Sthira*) Vishnuic, and the

---

* The terms *Cardinal*, *Fixed* and *Mutable* are preferred throughout this series of manuals, partly for the sake of uniformity and partly for other reasons.

common or Mutable (*Dwiswabhava*—double-natured—
Ubhaya) Iswaric.

The Cardinal signs mark the Sun's equinoxes and
solstices. They are equivalent to the "angular" houses
of the scheme of nativity, 1, 4, 7, and 10, and imply
prominence, power, height. The Fixed signs are
equivalent to the succedent houses, and imply support,
conservation, solidarity. The Mutable are indentified
with the cadent houses and signify submission, media-
tion, mutation. As we recede or fall from the angles
there comes a secession from power and prominence.
And so we find that those people born under cardinal
signs, or having many planets therein, possess a craving
for publicity, and incline to political and public offices.
Those under fixed signs somewhat less so, having, too,
more gravity, ballast and placidity, and gravitating to
those positions where firmness, stability, authority, are
requisite. While those under common signs are least
desirous of prominence, or if desirous, find it difficult to
acquire the realisation of such ambition, love the quiet
ways, serving, acting as mediator between the two
others, and generally obeying rather than commanding.

It must not be assumed from this that the power and
degree of morbid action will show a falling off from
cardinal to common ; that the intensity of disease will
be associated with the moveable, and its remission with
the mutational signs. Briefly, the necessity of considering this particular sign arrangement lies in the fact that
a mutual influence prevails among the members of each
of these three divisions. They are Mental (*cardinal*),
Vital (*fixed*), and Motive (*mutable*). The mutable or
common series of sympathetic co-ordinates is seen to
include the chief limb signs, and the fixed the heart and
generative ones. The temperamental trigons are so
constituted that a representative of each quaternion is

included.   In the fiery trigon for example, Aries belongs to the mental, Leo to the vital, and Sagittarius to the motive.   We have to meet the effects of this sympathy so frequently in the horoscopical deduction of disease tendencies, that we cannot do better than obtain early an appreciation of the inter-agency.

The three great aspects of especial pathologic effect are the conjunction (☌), quartile (□), and opposition (☍).   These are related to each other as :—the sign itself ; the immediate proximate and ultimate positional signs (that is the nearest sign of its own name—cardinal, fixed or mutable—preceding and succeeding) ; and the sign diametrically opposite, which also will be of the same name.   In this wise the four signs of any one series all become implicated.

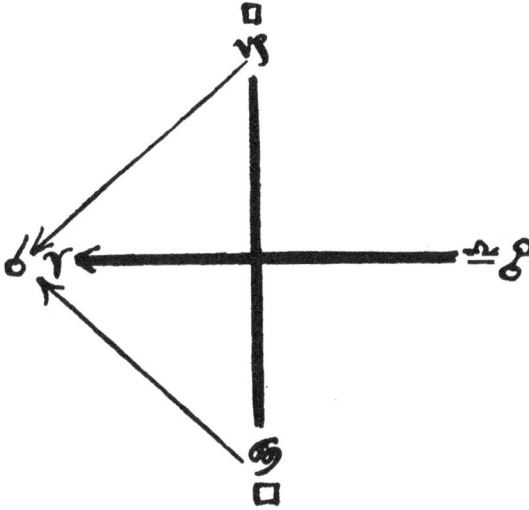

In illustration suppose we take the cardinal Aries,— then the cardinal signs on either side will be Cancer (succeeding), and Capricorn (preceding), while the oppositional division will be Libra. They were related to Aries (♂), as dexter (♑) and sinister (♋) squares (□), and opposition (☍). The four signs are thus held in a sort of mutual bondage.

The Hindu astrologer speaks of this oppositional aspect as a "full sight," because the points concerned, being 180 degrees apart, are *en regard*, the rays of two bodies so posited falling fully on each other; the quartile is the "three-quarter-sight."* The conjunction, of course, is not an aspect in reality, but a position, or as often expressed "the body." From this relationship there ensue a coanimity of parts and an interchange of forces. It will therefore be remarked that in those cases where cardinal signs are well tenanted, head, stomach, kidney and skin disorders will show themselves, although possibly Aries contains no planet; where fixed signs are occupied, maladies of the heart, throat, back and generative organs will occur; and where mutable signs, affections of the respiratory system, nerves and bowels. But while this is so, no sign loses altogether its distinctive value.

* For Mars, however, it is supposed to be a " full sight."

CHAPTER X.

Planetary Sympathy and Antipathy.

Towards the enucleation of this matter we must run over the fundamental properties of the planets, considering them from the vantage point of the *primum calidum*.

Heat and cold are related as drought and moisture, and though it is customary to refer to them as elemental qualities, that is not a true definition. Each celestial body differs from its compeers in the commingling of heat or cold with drought or moisture. The proportions are discovered by observing the affinity shown with sub-lunar matters. They may be expressed as below, the plus (+) sign being employed to denote the intense degree, and the minus (−) the remiss.

+ −	− +	+ +
⊙ Hot and dry	☽ Cold and moist	♄ Cold and dry
♃ Hot and moist	☿ Cold and dry (*con-*	− −
♄ Cold and dry	*vertible by aspect*)	ψ Warm and moist
	♀ Warm and moist	
	♂ Hot and dry	

However, it is only fair to state that Ptolemy and many others after him, accounted the Sun to possess moderate warmth and dryness (μετρίως ποιητικὴ δερμότητος, etc.); the Moon to be moist with a little warmth (τὸ πλεῖστον ὑγραντικὴ—μετέχει δὲ μετρίως θερμότητος); Mercury indifferent as to moisture and drought, sometimes one, sometimes the other (ἐξ ἴσου πότε μὲν ξηραίνει, πότε δὲ ‘υγραίνει); but yet on the whole rather dry (ὑπόξηρος);

57

Venus temperate, differing from Jupiter only in this respect: that while Jupiter inclines more to warmth than moisture, Venus is more moist than warm (τὴν αὐτήν ἔχει εὐκρασιαν, etc.); Mars, hot, dry and burning (καυστικός· δια τὸ πυρῶδες αυτου); Jupiter temperately warm and moist (θερμίνει ʽαμα καὶ ʽυγραίνει, ἀλλὰ τὸ πλέου ʺεχει τὸ θερμὸν, etc.); Saturn, cold and dry, but partaking more of the former than the latter quality (τὸ μὲν ψυχρὸν πλέον ʺεχει, τὸ δὲ ξηρὸν μετριώτερον).

Now heat will express itself as expansion, vitalisation; cold as contraction, crystallisation, and concretion; dryness as radiation, irritation; moisture as relaxation, mobility, plasticity. Admixtures will produce results in accordance. For example, the coalition of Moon and Mars will be equivalent to that of fire and water. Each will strive to subdue the other, the outcome being ebullition, evaporation, steam, conversion into an aëriform state, in the latter case; in the human organism, effervescent mental activity, displays of angry feeling, dispersal and dissipation of brain force, eruptive conditions. On the other hand there is an affinity between Mercury and Saturn, both possessing similar qualities, although in contrary proportions. Venus sympathises with Neptune for the same reason, and also with Jupiter and the Moon. The lunar coldness is not that of Saturn. It is a neutral condition, and may for ordinary purposes be regarded as temperate.

Let us suppose Mars conjoined with some other body and deduce the character of the resultant force in various spheres of activity. First with Jupiter. Both have points of agreement in being hot, but then Jupiter brings some moisture and Mars some dryness, and the dryness is seen by the table to be in greater degree than the humidity. We may illustrate the action by likening it to the operation of heat upon such substances as gums,

balsams, resins, sugar and the like. At first there is
the melting, accompanied by evaporation and inspissa-
tion, until the whole of the moisture has been driven
off; the solid residue ultimately chars. But if Saturn
take the place of Jupiter we shall represent the action
of the two by subjecting a piece of stone to the fire. In
this case melting does not occur; the stone flies abroad
in a thousand particles. The saturnine cold and the
martial heat are the extremes of negative and positive.
Even if otherwise, their dynamic action is too much at
variance to reconcile one with the other. In the domain
of disease Mars with Jupiter will increase the consistency
of adipose tissue and the connecting fibre. Mars with
Saturn will produce compound fractures, rapid extremes
of temperature, violent dispersals, etc. The action
may be likened to contending parties in a panic or crush,
one striving against the other, the upshot being a
catastrophe.

The combination of two planetary bodies whose
distinguishing properties are heat—such as Sun and
Mars—will enlarge the scope of diseases in which inflammatory and febrile symptoms are implicated. Con-
trariwise, where the attributes are conflicting—as in
Sun and Saturn—some minimising of each other's action
will eventuate. The solar inflammatory action will be
of the chronic type. The saturnine force will tend to
the devitalisation of the Sun's influence. A pair of
planets whose nature is cold and dry—such as Mercury
and Saturn—will be responsible for nervousness and
mental sagacity; when the dry predominates over the
cold—as in Mercury and Uranus—rapidity of thought,
exuberance of ideas, tangential moods and methods of
expression follow. And so with others.

A typical contrast is that of Mars and Saturn, and as
these two bodies are such prominent factors in the production of lesions and physiological derangements, a

further short review may be made as an addition to
what has already been advanced.

Just as surely as Mars enhances, Saturn depresses.
" Saturn," says Cardan, " causes long diseases, Mercury
various ones, the Moon such as return after a time, like
vertigo, epilepsy, etc., Jupiter and Sun short diseases,
but Mars the acutest of all." The two bodies here
particularised are *anaretic* or destructive to life, but in
far different ways. They represent extreme heat,
(solar heat specialised through Mars, and really the
more intensive, so far as we are concerned here) ; and
extreme cold. The force of heat is the expansion or
life of matter ; that of cold and gravity the contraction
or death. Their specific colours are red and blue
respectively. Sensitive plants like the mimosa grow
ten or a dozen times higher under red glass than under
blue. Plants, in fact, nurtured under glass of the latter
colour are weak and stunted in growth. The melancholic man subjected to the same conditions, feels his
spirits raised under the red rays, while the violent and
paroxysmic type is calmed and soothed under the blue.
The Mars lunatic will be violent, the Saturnine
hypochondriac.

Timidity and depression are Saturnine. In this
manner the orb acts as a restrictor, quite the opposite
of the expansive, frank Mars. The latter does not
make philosophers but men of action and impulse.
Timidity, or in another word Saturn, conduces to
meditation and analysis. The temperament of the
philosopher and scientist is bathed in it as, *per contra*,
that of the energetic pioneer is in Mars. In the
sedentary, intellectual man there is usually a great deal
of Saturn and very little of Mars ; or to put the same thing
another way : much speculative hardihood but little
practical and physical courage ; wisdom, but want of

" snap," mental perseverance and penetrativeness but dread of the crowd—*agoraphobia*—and dislike of physical activity. In the saturnine individual the mental consciousness is large, and takes precedence ; in the martial the animal soul is dominant. The one has a thin watery blood, the other a thick, rich, vital fluid, neither conducive to meditation nor inspiration, but to sensation and expiration. To understand this antithesis and to bring the facts well home it is only necessary to compare a series of horoscopes belonging to philosophers and scientists, with those of fighters and men of action.

To Mars are referable cases of determination of blood by the application of stimuli. Heat will cause a flow of blood to the surface, snuff to the nose and eyes, spices, etc., to the salivary glands, food to the secernent vessels, purgatives to those of the intestines, diuretics to those of the kidneys. And this brings us to the therapeutic treatment of disease by antipathetic remedies—the *contraria contraiis curantur* principle. *In exemplo*, the typical medicinal tonic—iron—is a remedy under Mars, something required by the blood in cases of want of tone, depression or flabbiness of the muscular system. In weak, lax habits, chronic disorders proceeding from debility, cachexy, hypochondriasis, in a word Saturnine complaints, ferrum is a stock remedy. It acts by quickening the circulation, raising the pulse, increasing the red particles of the blood and promoting the secretions. On the other hand antimony, a saturnine drug, operates in reducing fevers and inflammations, that is martial action. It is a contra-stimulant, diminishing the excitability of the vascular system, and so neutralising inflammatory conditions. Again, mark what happens upon the introduction of lead (♄) (in the form of salts) into the system. Exactly the opposite effects ensue to the exhibition of iron (♂), constipation, colic, tremors and resolutions of the nerves, contractions of the limbs, paralysis, atrophy, gout, etc., all representative saturnine disorders.   But almost as a last resource a preparation of lead (*Tinct. saturnina*) has been given for restraining the colliquative sweats in phthisis and hectic fevers.   Externally sugar of lead is used as an astrictive in collyria for inflammations of the eyes, as principal ingredient in unguents and liniments for cutaneous eruptions, excoriations, ulcers, etc.; and in the form of injections for restraining gonorrhœas. Saturnine remedies are in a peculiar manner injurious to the nervous system, over which Saturn exercises considerable influence.   Then, too, the operation of cold as a cause of disease by constricting the vessels of the surface and extremities, throwing the blood inwards, and producing internal congestions by intropulsion is diametrically opposed to the operations of Mars as illustrated by heat.   The veins and cutis, which contract with cold (♄), are relaxed with heat (♂).   A hæmorrhage (♂) will require a styptic (♄).   An inflammation or vascular excitement of the nervous centres (♂) an antiphlogistic (♄).   Deficiency of circulation in a part (♄) demands stimulant applications and friction, or perhaps internally strychnine or cantharides (♂).   Such affections as neuralgia when depending on a weak circulation (♄) are removed by tonics (♂).   Excessive voluntary power (♂) will require antimony, cold to the head, etc. (♄). And similarly in other cases.

The therapeutic side of astrology is very much undeveloped, but the course to follow is plainly indicated. As Paracelsus wrote: " The sympathy between planet and planet, so easy of observation, is a proof of the diffusion of collateral elements throughout the various channels of expression and of a constant stream of influences for ever interacting between those that stand thus related to each other.   Every metal and every plant possesses certain qualities that may attract corresponding planetary influences, and if we know the influences of the stars, the conjunctions of the planets and the qualities of drugs, we shall know what remedies to give to attract such influence as may act beneficially upon the patient."   Some typical drugs and "simples" will be found in Chapter V. together with the planetary powers to which they are allied.   This is the most that can be done in the way of *materia medica* so far as the present chapters are concerned.

Hitherto, the aspects and combinations of planets have been chiefly those in which the luminaries, the ascendant and some other body have been concerned. Yet aspects form between planets proper and exercise specific influences.   These will have to be gauged by the light of what information has been previously imparted.   However, the effects of the two bodies to which this chapter is mainly devoted may be briefly summarised.

By being *with* a planet is here meant, either the actual conjunction itself, or some aspect based on the square and not on the trine.

MARS WITH

SUN.—Increases the susceptibility to feverish, inflammatory and hyperæmic action.   High temperature, rapid pulse, excessive voluntary power.

MOON.—Copious menstrual discharges.   Pyrosis, bilious nausea and eructations.   Exanthematous fevers, eruptive action.

MERCURY.—Irritates the nervous system,—excitability, logorrhœa, etc., as pathogenic signs.   Nerve inflammation, erethism of nervous centres.   Bilious diarrhœa, neuroma, thirst.

VENUS.—Copious urinal discharge, excessive secretions, renal irritation, fibroma, phlebitis, nymphomania (in females),

JUPITER.—Lipoma, arthritis, fibrinous exudations, steatomatous tumour, adipose sarcoma, sthenic inflammation.

SATURN.—Biliary calculi, inflammation in joints, malformations, fractures, achondroplasia, according to which is the dominant planet.

URANUS.—Pains and cramps from exalted excitomotory function, involuntary muscular excitement, hyperkinetic action, lacerations and ruptures.

NEPTUNE.—Phenomena referable to psychic causes.

SATURN WITH

SUN.—Locomotory and spinal defects, lowered vitality, paralysis, heart and spinal centres affected, rigor, diseased voluntary power, lesions of the motory columns within the spine, structural diseases of heart, deep-seated complaints.

MOON.—Anæmic, narrow chested, cachectic, impaired sensorial functions, encephalic and intropulsive congestion, maturation and softening of tubercle.

MERCURY.—Deficient secretion of mucus on respiratory membrane, numbness of nerve.

VENUS.—Highly loaded urine, urinary calculi, suppression of urine.*

MARS.—Biliary calculi, inflammation in joints, malformations, fractures, achondroplasia, according to which is the dominant planet.

JUPITER.—Chondroma *(fibrocartilaginous tumour)*, sluggish liver, congestive inflammation if Jupiter the more dominant.

URANUS.—Contortion of rigid parts, compression of organs, contractions and strictures.

NEPTUNE.—Obscure and psychic.

---

* Placidus gives an instance of *retention* of urine, which was probably a *suppression*, in the horoscope of the Duchess of Sfortia, who is related to have died from the former cause.   Venus was in the sixth house in par. dec. with Saturn in Libra.

CHAPTER XI.

Gauging Planetary Strength in the Specific Horoscope.

However intimately we may be acquainted with the intrinsic virtues of members of the solar system, the knowledge will only avail us to a limited extent. We have now to draw in the threads so as to finally adjust and tighten up the whole scheme. It remains for us to consider in order what increase or surcease of vivific and morbific energy is induced by the aspects, and the actual planetary location in points of the natal chart. Planetary influence in the zodiacal hierarchies has already been considered in Chapter VII.

In sloka (*distich*) 38 of the Jataka Parijata six kinds of strength are enumerated:

> *Drikbalam.*—Strength of aspect.
> *Sthanabalam.*—Strength of position.
> *Nisargikabalam.*—Natural strength.
> *Cheshtabalam.*—Motional strength.
> *Dikbalam.*—Directional strength
> *Kalabalam.*—Temporal strength.

As an instance of the application of these arguments, let us take the positional strength (*sthanabalam*) of a planet. The following locations have jointly to be considered :

1. *Atchi Ucha*, or greatest exaltation.
2. *Ucha*, or exaltation.
3. *Mulatrikona*, or special house of power.
4. *Svakshetra*, or own house.
5. *Atimitra*, or very friendly house.
6. *Mitra*, or friendly house.
7. *Sama*, or neutral house.
8. *Satru*, or inimical house.
9. *Atisatru*, or very inimical house.
10. *Muda*, or combust.
11. *Nicha*, or house of debility.
12. *Atinicha*, or house of greatest debility.

The conception is of too colossal proportions for our Western ideas, yet it is very much akin to what will be here advanced. For before we are able to arrive at a judgment we shall have to consider (1) an aspect strength, (2) a strength of mundane position, (3) a natural strength, (4) a motional strength, and (5) a directional strength.

(1) Aspect Strength.

It is assumed that the reader is familiar with the aspects, their number of degrees and constitutional quality. We shall employ these :

EVIL				INTERDEPENDENT			GOOD	
Opposit.	*Quincunx*	*Quartile*	*Semiquartile*	*Par. dec.*		*Conj.*	*Trine*	*Sextile*
180°	150°	90°	45°				120°	60°
☍	⊼	□	∠	‖ or P.		☌	△	✳

The parallel of declination and conjunction or " body " are, generally speaking, good with good planets, evil with the reverse. On the left are the " goats " ; to the right the " lambs."

At first sight it seems inconceivable that evil factors like Mars and Saturn, or benefic ones like Venus and

Jupiter, should have their qualities so modified through being posited at various degrees apart, that the influence of the former should become a constructive instead of a destructive agency, and the latter the reverse. It is one of the objections urged by Plotinus. For a planet to change its nature by mere change of place or aspect was, he argued, so contrary to what happened in the sub-lunar sphere, that reasoning by analogy it could not be admitted. "The instability existing among the planets," he says, "can be inferred when each change in the form of an aspect is accompanied also by a change in its influence, as the astrologers affirm." In the third book of the second Ennead under the heading of Του ει ποιει τα αστρα he observes that "they [*the planets*] are adjudged to change their signification by their change of course, and as they are located in angles or cadent therefrom. But the most important thing they [*the astrologers*] say is that some among them are benefic, others evil, yet nevertheless the latter often perform as though endowed with the virtue of the former, no less than the former sometimes acting as the latter. They add that when the planets are in reciprocal aspect they act in one way, and when they do not aspect each other they produce effects in another. . . Lastly, a planet aspected by a certain favourable one bestows good, only to be suddenly changed when it transfers its aspect to another. They affirm likewise that they are changed in a certain manner according as the figure of aspecting is changed, and that from the body or mutual conjunction still another form of influence is generated."

In reality, the stars do not change their nature by change of position and configuration as asserted; nor are some good, others evil. In themselves they are neither. What happens is a fresh polarisation, a re-

arrangement of the energic rays.   Mars is always Mars;
it never exhibits the qualities of Saturn, nor presents
itself in the form of the latter—coldness, gravity, concretion.   But it cannot be gainsaid that the human
organism is adversely affected when receiving rays
through the medium of any of the evil aspects, even
when the planetary bodies involved are otherwise beneficial; much more so when the combined forces are
malefic.

It thus becomes imperative to accept a division of
the stars into malefic and benefic, and to assume that
there is an inherent capability among them for mutual
mingling and transference of influence.   Theoretically
the explanation is not so difficult, but we are dealing
with facts here.   Let us therefore think of each separate
influence as having a functioning potentiality of two
phases: (a) an *anabolismic* or life-force producing, and (b)
a *katabolismic* or life-force destroying.   The former will
manifest under the series of aspects based on the
triangle; the latter under those based on the square.
Thus, Sun trine Mars (☉ △ ♂) will give the best, the
constructive form of martial influence, and that which
is directly beneficial to mankind.   There will result
stamina of body, activity, great energy, will power,
force of character, ability to lead and control, to upbuild
and act with promptitude, courage and dispatch.   Sun
quartile Mars (☉ □ ♂) however, will show the other
side of the medal.   Here we still have activity, energy,
force of character, etc., but the nature of the person
will possess the dark traits of the planet—anger,
passional violence, vindictiveness.   It will destroy
rather than build, inflame rather than produce a cherishing warmth, and provide all the requisite conditions for
inflammatory and febrile action.   In both cases the
force of the planet is expressed through the Sun, and

as both bodies are positive, electric and caloric-producing, it is easily seen that in the latter instance diseases will be acute, violent, feverish, excessive, poignant and inflammatory. Such injuries and complaints will ensue as cause loss of blood, surgical operations, wounds by edged tools, gun-shots, burns, scalds. Injuries and disorders will proceed from rash and self-motived acts, and may vary according to the state of the horoscope as a whole, from hurts by accident to suicide or assassination. For these latter come within the purview of astrology, being associated with the disorganisation expressed through the stars just as much as the actual morbific predisposition.

The aspecting angles* which exert most power are the conjunction, par. dec., quartile and opposition. The conjunction is not so unbalancing as the square and opposition; and whereas the previously mentioned trine of Mars to the Sun is wholly constructive, presenting the very best attributes of Mars, and the square or opposition on the other hand wholly destructive, the conjunction possesses in a large measure the capacities of each and will function at different times in either manner. If well supported the worst need not be feared. Still, the balance will always incline to the wrong side.

It is evident that the greater the number of these evil aspects received by the luminaries the more will the organism be predisposed to disorder; while the more malefic the aspecting bodies and the completer the angles of aspects themselves, the more profound will such disorder be.

---

* The word 'angles' is here used in its usual geometric sense, but it may be well to remind the reader of its technical astrological usage as an abbreviation for 'angular houses,' namely houses 1, 4, 7, 10.

Also, we see, if we have placed in our hands merely the planetary data, we are enabled at once to cognise the diathesis—on broad lines, of course. That is to say, if we are told there is heavy saturnine affliction we understand there will be a susceptibility to cold, chronic, tedious, consumptive, corruptive, obstructive disorders. If Uranus, nervous, spasmodic, neuralgic maladies. If Mars, inflammatory, feverish, acute, contagious, violent and sudden complaints. And so with others.

But this definite expression of some dominant planet is by no means an invariable circumstance. It is readily conceivable that a mingling of various forces may prevail, and in the disentangling of these the difficulty lies. There is all the difference as between an elementary atom and a compound molecule.

Now the explanation usually afforded by chemistry in regard to the combination of atoms is based upon the assumption that each atom has a certain definite number of bonds, or poles, analogous to those of the magnet. This quality is known as quantivalence, and an atom may be univalent, bivalent, quinquivalent, etc. If we think of the planetary bodies in a similar sense, (and simply as an illustrative conception), we shall take them as the atoms and their quantivalence will be represented by their aspects. And so if in any horoscope we were confronted with a scheme of solar aspects such as the following : ⊙ □ ♄, ∠ ♆, ☌ ♅, ☍ ♂ , we obtain a quadrivalent quantivalence for the Sun, thus :—

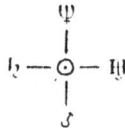

$$\begin{array}{c} ♆ \\ | \\ ♄ - \odot - ♅ \\ | \\ ♂ \end{array}$$

and if at the same time Mars aspects Saturn ; Mercury,

Mars and Saturn; and Uranus, Neptune; the further complications will be indicated by other *vinculi*, thus:—

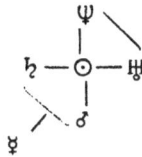

$$\begin{array}{c}\Psi\\ | \quad \backslash \\ \hbar - \odot - \Hull \\ \diagdown \quad | \\ \diagup \cdot \, \delta \\ \breve\end{array}$$

(2) MUNDANE STRENGTH.

This depends upon the character of that division of a natal scheme wherein any planet-star happens to be posited.

The angles are undoubtedly the pre-eminent points, and the action of those bodies which occupy ascendant, occident, medium cœli and imum cœli is increased in a remarkable way. There are two other houses which have special significance in disease, *viz.*, the sixth and twelfth; but of their dominion we shall see more in Chapter VIII. The third and ninth houses are also important, since they are concerned with the mind, and mental conditions are responsible for a physical reflection. For the rest, a planet gains in strength and potency by being elevated above its fellows.

It must be borne in mind that the twelve mundane divisions, the *templa, regiones*, or *mansiones* of the geniture, commonly known as the Twelve Houses, are the equivalent of the celestial zodiac. They are the co-significators of the signs.*

---

* As this book is likely to be read by many who have no previous acquaintance with the technology of the subject we trust we may be excused for directing the reader's attention specially to this paragraph. The mutual correspondence of the *houses* and the *signs*, and the unfortunate use by many writers of the word "house"

The first house (*see the Example Horoscope given on
p. 78*) has a similar meaning to the first sign Aries, the
second to Taurus, the third to Gemini, and so on.
Their powers from a physiological point of view,
however, are much less extensive—except in the case
of angles; the Eastern corresponding to Aries, the
Northern to Cancer, the Western to Libra and the
Southern to Capricorn.   But of special moment is
the first named—the ascendant—and evil planetary
activity here is always extremely liable to find a morbid
outlet on the material plane through the head itself.   But
with the remaining houses no testimony must be accepted
unsupported by zodiacal endorsement, unless a stellium
of planets gives more than ordinary importance to a
house.   For example, suppose in a geniture the fifth
house were heavily tenanted, then the heart and back
would be likely to suffer, although the actual cardiac
sign Leo might be unoccupied.   The determination
would be strengthened and accentuated if the sign
containing the affliction in the fifth were of fixed quality.
Similarly an over-cargo in the second house would react
upon the throat; in the third, upon the lungs and nerves,
arms or hands; in the fourth, upon the stomach, etc.

---

to signify a sign of the zodiac rather than a one-twelfth-part of
the mundane sphere, is the cause of much confusion of thought
among those just commencing the study of astrology—a confusion
which need never arise if sufficient emphasis is laid upon the
distinction at the start.   The complications resulting from the
interplay of these two series, *houses* and *signs*, may be more easily
imagined than enumerated.   Thus, if Libra ascend, and Mars be
placed in Aries in the seventh house, then the natural Seventh
House is in the mundane position of the First House, while the
ruler of the natural First is in the actual Seventh.   This inter-
relationship is entered into more fully in the Introductory Manual
of this series, and the simile there made use of in reference to it
will perhaps be found helpful.

(3) NATURAL STRENGTH.

The natural strength arises from the sympathy or antipathy which exists between the planet and the sign it occupies. It will be strongest in its own sign and in those signs most compatible with its nature. But from our point of view it will work most havoc when occupying signs with which it has no affinity, thereby setting up discord and producing disorganisation. For instance, a fiery planet will be out of its element in watery signs, while a humid one such as the Moon will not be disposed to associate favourably with fiery signs.

And here may be introduced a doctrine not much regarded by modern astrologers, but yet one which exhibits a phase of planetary activity by interchange that is of considerable importance in numbers of cases which otherwise, *i.e.*, without the explanation it affords, would be deemed irregular. I allude to planetary reception by sign. This happens when a couple of bodies occupy signs each of which is the proper sign of the other. If Mars is in Cancer and the Moon in Aries reception takes place. In this instance it is of very evil augury. Each is usurping the natural place of the other and neither has affinity with the sign it actually tenants. But the matter does not rest here. Its utility lies in the individual application, and goes far to explain many seeming irregularities. Take the Soli-Saturnian influence. Three allied forms of this will be manifest: the aspect influence (say ☉ ☌ ♄); Sun in Capricorn; and Saturn in Leo. The admixtures will of course vary in intensity, but there is a thread of connection common to them all. A table as below will show at a glance the receptions by house of the luminaries. Tables for the other planets may easily be constructed on the same plan.

SUN.   MOON.

$$\odot \text{ in } \begin{cases} \text{♈ ♏} - \text{♂} \\ \text{♉ ♎} - \text{♀} \\ \text{♊ ♍} - \text{☿} \\ \text{♋} - \text{☽} \\ \text{♐} - \text{♃} \\ \text{♑} - \text{♄} \\ \text{♒} - \text{♅} \\ \text{♓} - \text{♇} \end{cases} \text{ in ♌} \qquad \text{☽ in } \begin{cases} \text{♈ ♏} - \text{♂} \\ \text{♉ ♎} - \text{♀} \\ \text{♊ ♍} - \text{☿} \\ \text{♌} - \text{☉} \\ \text{♐} - \text{♃} \\ \text{♑} - \text{♄} \\ \text{♒} - \text{♅} \\ \text{♓} - \text{♇} \end{cases} \text{ in ♋}$$

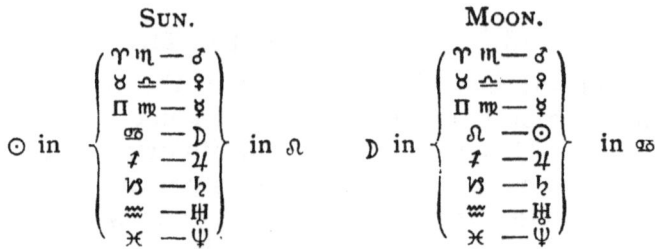

(4) MOTIONAL STRENGTH.

Under this heading are included (a) the actual rate of longitudinal motion of any planet, (b) its retrogradation, (c) its stationary attitude. The daily rate of zodiacal progression varies within certain limits, and consequently when the 'tempo' is slow the application and resolution of aspects are more protracted and likely to occasion a greater degree of disturbance in the physical organism. The mean daily motion of the various planets is as follows : Neptune about $\frac{1}{2}'$, Uranus slightly less than 1', Saturn 2', Jupiter 5', Mars 33'28", Sun, Mercury and Venus 59', Moon 13°10'. Motion is slow or quick as it falls short or exceeds this mean. Retrograde motion, although only an apparent phenomenon, may yet produce some amount of disorganisation even if only because a planet retrograde is then nearest the earth. It implies interrupted sequence, solution of continuity, just as direct motion does continuity and sequence of progression. The writer has noticed that a retrograde Jupiter is robbed of much of its supporting power and cannot be depended upon to sustain life when evil directions are formed. The stationary position of a planet indicates constancy and duration of effects ; bodies therefore have the sphere of their influence enlarged according as their intrinsic nature warrants, i.e., benefic or malefic. " It would not be easy," says Wilson, "to demonstrate why the motion of a planet, whether swift or slow, direct or retrograde, should alter its influence, which must wholly proceed from attraction." On the whole, motional strength is rather an uncertain factor, or at least we have not sufficient data to go upon so far as the question of disease is implicated.

(5) DIRECTIONAL STRENGTH.

This is the power of planets holding each other in aspect at a period subsequent to birth.* The various bodies have moved forward in the zodiac and through the houses of the scheme, and as fresh arrangements and admixtures of rays are effected a ready responsion is made by the human organism. The "direction" will indicate both type and time of disease, but only that will be consummated which is foreshadowed in the radix (it is very important to remember this).

The directional strength must therefore depend upon a combination of the foregoing, *viz.*, aspect, mundane position, zodiacal location.

There is a *hexis* or permanent habit as well as a *diathesis* or transient disposition. The hexis is shown in the *radix*, the diathesis in the *direction*. If the diathesis agree with the hexis the disorder indicated is more certain and pronounced: that is to say if there is evil martial influence in the geniture the native will more readily respond to martial directions, and suffer from or succumb to inflammatory, acute, or febrile disease, be subjected to violence or undergo surgical operations. If Saturnine influence, then chronic and cachectic types. Similarly with others.

---

* For complete exposition and method see the Manual *Directions and Directing*, also *The Progressed Horoscope*.

CHAPTER XII.

APPLICATION.

WE have gathered that the planets under certain circumstances are inimical to mankind, and that among them some are more virulent than others. Indeed while we regard one contingent as 'aphetic' or life protecting and cherishing, another is just as surely 'anaretic' or life destroying.

And so it comes about that representatives of this latter—Mars, Saturn, Uranus—are the more imperative factors in the production of disease and death. (Not that the other bodies are innoxious when their vibrations are disturbed by antipathetic confliction with others, but only that their malefic powers under such conditions do not reach so high a pitch as those of the bodies mentioned).

Also, we have realised that there are three vital centres—SUN, MOON, and ASCENDANT. Ptolemy, it is true, prescribed particular divisions of the ambient to be "prorogatory" or aphetic places, and that the occupation of such by one of the luminaries constituted that luminary the giver of life, death only ensuing under its affliction by direction. But his methods of deciding this point are too arbitrary to enlist unquestioning adherence, and in actual practice do not prove of much utility.

In every horoscope upon which judgment of disease has to be given, the following series of investigations must be instituted:

76

(1) To consider how and in what degree the three aphetic points, *Sun, Moon,* and *Ascendant,* are afflicted or preserved.

(2) The type of energy represented by the afflicting bodies.

(3) The strength of such bodies.

(4) The signification of the houses and signs occupied.

(5) The mutual affliction among planets, not involving the three centres of Sun, Moon and Ascendant.

It is obvious that there will be static points and kinetic points for each planet, the former represented by its longitudinal degree of location in a sign, the latter by the points to which aspects are thrown. But the place of the aspect must be met by a distributing force in the shape either of another planet or the cusp of the Ascendant, otherwise the influence is disseminated without any result upon the physical organism—that is, so far as the aspect-sign is concerned. As an example we will take a nativity.* (Page 78.)

---

* The ordinary circular map block will be familiar to most readers, doubtless, but for the sake of others it may be explained that the double lines represent the two great circles of the Meridian and Horizon respectively, the symbols and figures at their extremities showing the points of the zodiac (ecliptic) which they cut, at the moment of birth and in the latitude and longitude of the birth-place : they determine the " cusps " or boundary lines of the f ur " angular houses," or " angles," the 1st, 4th, 7th and 10th houses that is to say. The heavy numerals indicate that the spaces in which they are found comprise the houses severally designated by the numerals in question. The diagram represents the heavens as they would appear to an observer in the N. Hemisphere standing with his face to the South, the Ascendant or Rising Sign appearing in the East on his left, planets setting in the West towards his right, and those culminating near the Zenith and towards the South. Hence the position of the Sun at once gives a clue to the time of day for which the figure was cast.

HOROSCOPE OF A MALE CHILD.

Born July 4th, 1906, 2h. 40m. p.m   Lat. 52°30'N, Long.95°E.

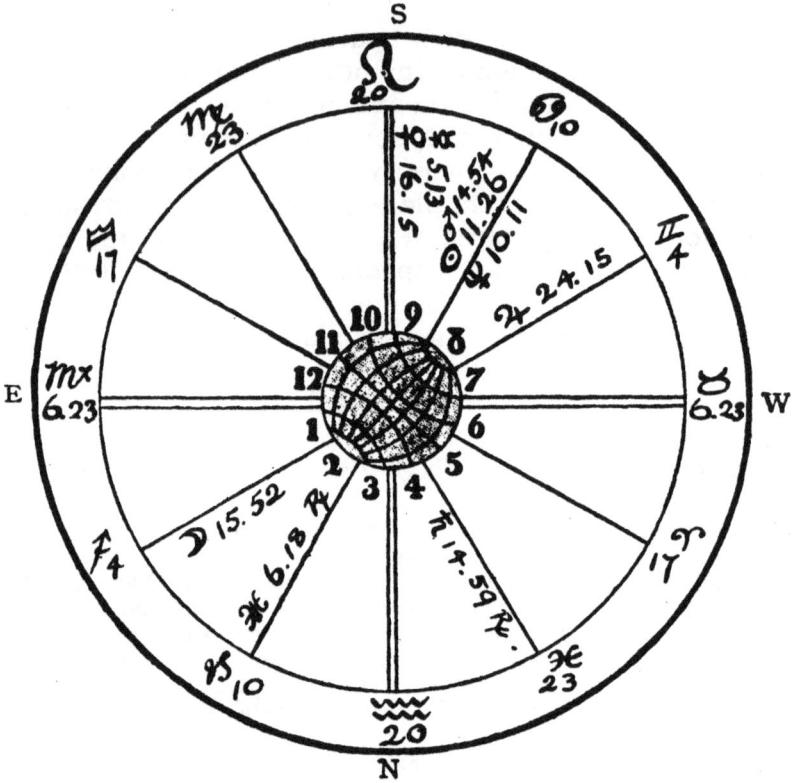

Declinations.

	° ′		° ′		° ′
☉	22 58 N	♀	17 40 N	♄	7 40 S
☽	18 20 S	♂	23 35 N	♅	23 37 S
☿	20 8 N	♃	22 58 N	♆	22 11 N

[See footnote on p. 77].

DISTRIBUTORY SCHEME.

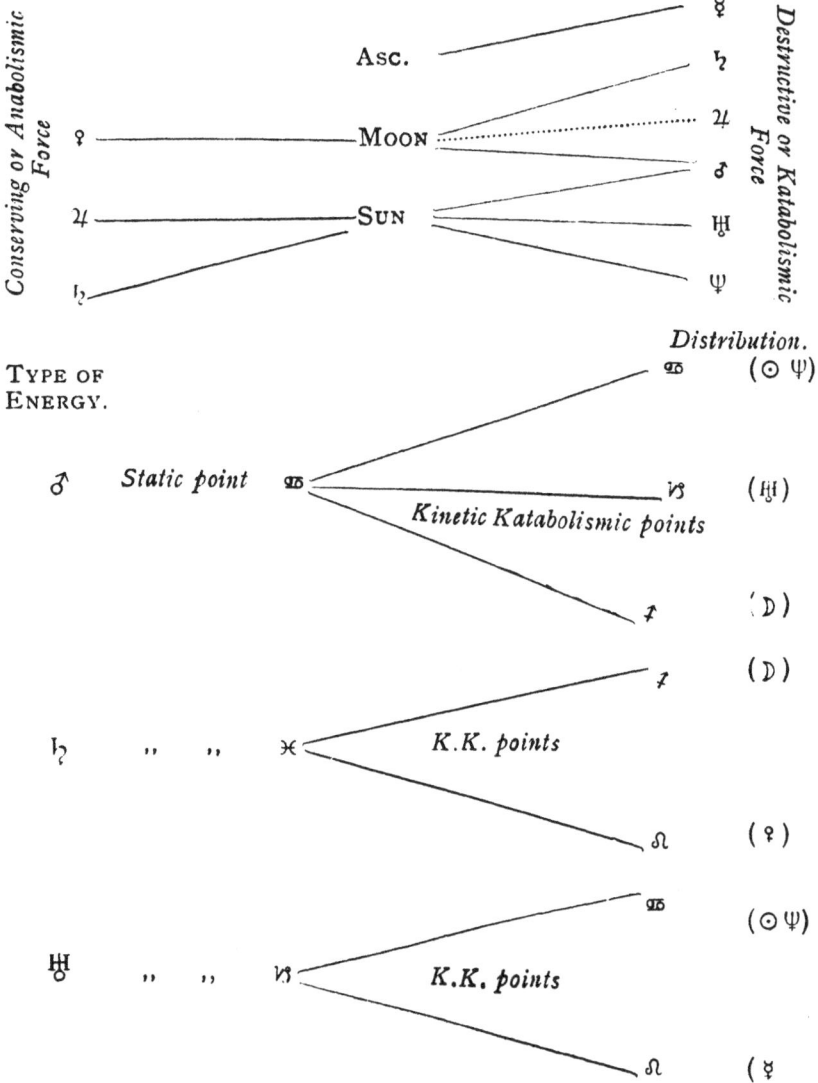

Planets in Signs.

	☽	♅		♄			♃	☉ ♂ Ψ	☿ ♀		
♏	♐	♑	♒	♓	♈	♉	♊	♋	♌	♍	♎
8th	9th	10th	11th	12th	Asc.	2nd	3rd	4th	5th	6th	7th
♃	Ψ' ♂ ☉ ☿	♀					☽	♅	♄		

Planets in Houses.

Here, by reference to the tables immediately succeeding the *thema cœli*, we first note (p. 79) a preponderance of katabolismic activity, and next we observe that on the other hand assistance is thrown from the opposite side through the medium of Venus, Jupiter and Saturn. By the instrumentality of these latter the life will gain in length and the system in recuperative power. Yet, although the native may appear robust, his constitution is delicate, for not only are the luminaries afflicted, *separatim*, but they are unfavourably related by the quincunxial aspect.

Underneath we observe the three worst types of destructive energy, and where they are functioning by body, and also to what points they are empowered to flash forth that energy. First we note Mars with a static position in Cancer and kinetic katabolismic poles in the same sign, Capricorn and Sagittarius, the distribution of the energy being among Sun and Neptune; Uranus; and Moon, respectively in these signs. This shows intense martial action. Secondly, Saturn static in Pisces, kinetic energy to Sagittarius (☾) and Leo (♀). This is a coagulating, depressing, cachectic influence. Finally, Uranus from Capricorn throws rays to Cancer (☉ ♅) and Leo (☿)—a perverting, disruptive agency. Thus while the Sun suffers from the Martial and Uranian radiations, the Moon receives the energies of Mars and Saturn, the former being elevated above the latter.

This implies that there is a lot of unbalanced force and vigour in the constitution, and that the pull of the activities involved will periodically result in disruptures. The organism, in fact, will be required to endure perverted tonic disorders mostly. The life-force will bubble up with such dynamic intensity as to come near effecting its own destruction.

The solar-martial action in Cancer will produce not only great irritability of stomach, with difficulty in retaining food (Byron had Mars in Cancer), but also hæmorrhage and acute gastritis. Neptune and Uranus being concerned too, indicate complications and obscure præincipients, perverted activity resulting in morbid growths, probably cancerous. Precautions should be taken in regard to malarial and camp fevers.

The third table (p. 80) compares and contrasts the planets' respective house- and sign-positions, and needs no comment.

Nervous and pulmonary complaints are betokened : (☾ in ♐ approaching opposition of ♃ in ♊). Pleurisy and intercostal neuralgia will also be experienced. The stomach, lungs and nerves are all marked by overactivity, and are here the great centres of disease. Death will be violent owing to the affliction of the luminaries by anaretic bodies,

F

CHAPTER XIII.

EXAMPLES.

SPACE can only be afforded for a few examples—and those of the more regular types, for unfortunately there are cases which exhibit at first sight many seemingly irregular features. The bare hints furnished in those ensuing should be supplemented by a detailed study of the figures themselves, erected from the elements given.

DIPHTHERIA.—This is an acute, infectious disease associated with a membranous exudation on a mucous surface, *viz.*, throat, tonsils or pharynx. It is chiefly identified with the fixed signs, but especially Taurus and Scorpio. Also, as isolation or detention in hospital is implied, the twelfth house is likely to be prominent, probably containing one of the luminaries or one of the afflicting bodies. The Moon is usually afflicted by Saturn and the Sun by Venus.

(1) *Female :* November 4th, 1895, 7.30 a.m., London. Here we have Scorpio rising with Mars, Saturn, Sun and Uranus—a terrible affliction. Mercury is on the cusp of twelfth, and Mars is well in same house. The Sun is conjoined with Saturn, Mars and Uranus. Moon is afflicted by Mars. The ominous state of affairs can be appreciated by a glance at the subpended diagram showing the twelfth and first houses;

XII.

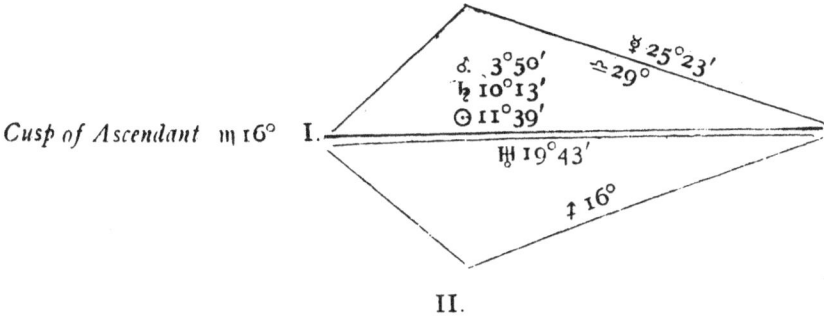

Cusp of Ascendant ♏ 16° I.

♂ 3°50'
♄ 10°13'
☉ 11°39'
☿ 25°23'
♎ 29°
♅ 19°43'
♐ 16°

II.

The child died November 4th, 1896.

(2) *Male* : April 26th, 1894, 6.45 a.m., Lat. 51°30'N., Long. 0°40'E. The Sun is in Taurus and the twelfth, opposed by Uranus and applying to a quartile of Mars and a semi-quartile of Venus. The Moon is in the eighth squared by Saturn and Mercury. Three bodies occupy fixed signs, three fixed houses.

(3) *Male* : October 12th, 1897, 8.45 a.m., Peckham. The signs Taurus and Scorpio are again involved. The

XII.

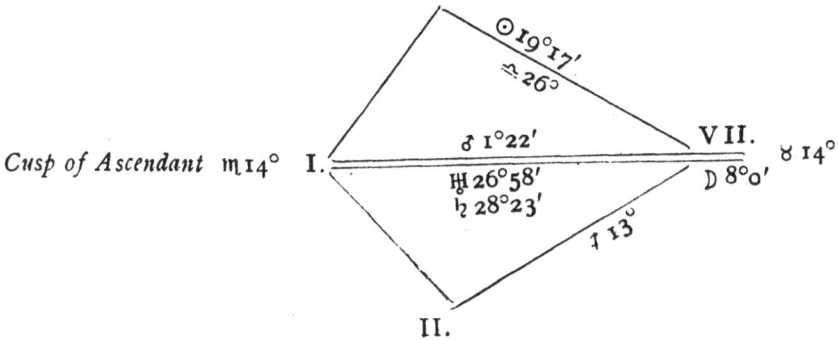

Cusp of Ascendant ♏ 14° I.

☉ 19°17'
♎ 26°
♂ 1°22'
♅ 26°58'
♄ 28°23'
VII.
♉ 14°
☽ 8°0'
♐ 13°

II.

Sun is on the twelfth house cusp and the Moon heavily oppressed on the seventh.

(4) *Female:* October 27th, 1891, 1 p.m., Lat. 40°0' N., Long. 85°12'W.* Here we still have Scorpio to the fore, providing house room for the Sun, Mercury, Venus and Uranus. The Moon is in Virgo receiving the square of Neptune and the opposition of Jupiter. But we must note that· the ascendant (♒1°0') has the squares from Sun, Mercury and Uranus, and that the malefics Mars and Saturn occupy the eighth house—a house we have learnt to associate with the zodiacal sign Scorpio. The child died when the Sun and· Mercury completed their quartile aspects to the ascending point. Some idea of the relationship can be gathered from the appended tabulation.

It is well· to note that a predisposing cause of diphtheria is scarlet fever, a complaint which is itself identified with Taurus and Scorpio.

---

* NOTE—In all cases the Standard Time in use at the birth‑place is to be presumed unless otherwise specified. For details as to Standards of Time in use in various parts of the world, consult *Casting the Horoscope.*

HIP-JOINT DISEASE.—Saturnine affliction in Sagittarius, either by actual location of the planet itself, or rays thrown to the Sun or other important body; Mars usually forms an aspect. Two characteristic examples follow:

(1) *Male :* December 3rd, 1868, 8.30 p.m., Lat. 41°52' N., Long. 87°35'W.

Ascendt.	☉	☽	☿	♀	♂	♃
♌6°	♐12°12'	♌4°15'	♏26°5'	♏5°10'	♌29°21'	♈4°20'

	♄	♅	♆
	♐8°41'	♋16°3'	♈14°42'

The Sun and Saturn are conjoined in Sagittarius, Mars is applying to the quartile of the solar orb, and the latter to the quincunx of Uranus.

(2) *Male:* November 22nd, 1853, 5.40 p.m., Lat. 53°23'N., Long. 10*m.* 12*s.*W.

Ascendt.	☉	☽	☿	♀	♂	♃
♋2°	♐0°23'	♌16°38'	♐20°38'	♑15°53'	♍2°41'	♐28°0'

	♄	♅	♆
	♉28°9'	♉9°48'	♓10°56'
	℞	℞	

Sagittarius is tenanted by the Sun, Mercury and Jupiter, these bodies being afflicted and in the sixth house of the scheme. The Sun receives the opposition of Saturn, quartiles of Neptune and Mars, and semi-quartile of Venus; Mercury and Jupiter have the quincunx of Saturn.

This was a case of spina bifida also. Observe Moon in Leo badly aspected by Uranus and Venus, and applying to the square of Saturn.

CONVULSIONS.—The factors in convulsions will be found to consist in (*a*) a preponderating number of planets in fixed signs; (*b*) the Moon, and generally

Mercury, receiving evil rays from Saturn and Uranus;
(c) the presence of the four bodies mentioned in Fixed
signs.   In serious cases resulting in death, of course,
the aspects are very pronounced.

(1) *Female :* January 16th, 1896, 3.5 p.m.* (died
November 27th, 1896).   Here we have five bodies in
fixed signs.   The Moon and Mercury in Aquarius are
squared by Saturn and· Uranus in Scorpio and opposed
by Jupiter in Leo.   There were croup and diphtheria too.

(2) *Male :* January 22nd, 1899, 9 a.m.————(died
March 28th, 1899).   This was a case of congestion of the
lungs attended by convulsions.   Five bodies are in lung
signs.   The Moon occupies Gemini and receives the
opposition of Saturn, Uranus and Venus, and the
conjunction of Neptune.   The Sun is afflicted by a
semi-quartile of Saturn, a quartile of Jupiter and an
opposition of Mars.

(3) *Female :* November 25th, 1894, 9.45 a.m.————
(died June, 1895.) Four bodies occupy the fixed sign
Scorpio—Moon, Mercury, Saturn and Uranus — in
mutual affliction, and receiving the rays of Neptune by
a quincunx.

DISEASES OF OR ACCIDENTS TO THE EYES.—The
luminaries are generally in mutual affliction, one of them
frequently rising, while Mars or Saturn throws a malefic
ray.   The worst signs for the luminaries in this respect
are Aries, Cancer, Taurus, Capricorn, Leo and Aquarius
—Taurus and Aquarius being especially constant.   It
is almost a matter of certainty to find the eyes suffering
when an afflicted Moon is located in either of these latter.

---

* Here and elsewhere, where place of birth is not stated
(indicated by dash) it has either not been communicated or is
withheld in deference to native's desire; it may be presumed as
within the British Isles in all cases.

If Uranus, Saturn, or Mars afflict, and the Moon is in the first, fourth or seventh decreasing in light, total blindness often occurs. Mars will cause blindness by fire, explosion, gunshot, lightning, wounds, smallpox; Saturn by colds, cataracts, specks, etc.; Mercury from eye-strain due to hard reading, mental exertion, etc. The Sun afflicted in ascendant is liable to cause cataract.

(1) *Female:* July 9th, 1884, 4.26 a.m., Lat. 52°28′N., Long. 7*m*. W.

Ascendt.	☉	☽	☿	♀	♂	♃
♋23°	♋17°18′	♑26°1′	♒12°27′	♋21°53′ ℞	♍19°27′	♌9°9′

	♄	♅	♆
	♊18°7′	♏24°40′	♉22°44′

This scheme shows the Sun rising, opposed by a decreasing Moon in the seventh, the signs involved being Cancer and Capricorn. Four planets and the ascendant are in these signs. Extreme myopia and astigmatism.

(2) *Female:* July 13th, 1853, noon. Birthplace not stated. (*Modern Astrology*, Vol. II., Old Series, p. 43.) Blind. Here the Moon rises in Libra in quartile to a culminating Sun in Cancer. The Moon is heavily afflicted by a sesquiquadrate of Saturn (in Taurus), and a quincunx of Uranus (also in Taurus).

(3) *Male:* June 27th, 1887, 10.40 a.m., Lat. 50°44′N., Long. 1°50′W. The Moon rises in the end of Virgo in square to Mars and Sun, and applying to the conjunction of Uranus. Myopia.

(4) *Male:* September 12th, 1875, 5 p.m., Lat. 45°N., Long. 0°12′E. The Moon is rising conjoined with Saturn and opposed by Uranus from Leo. The Sun is in seventh. Blind from birth.

Cases in which one or both of the luminaries are located and afflicted in Taurus: *Male:* January 22nd,

1888, 4.30 p.m.————(going blind). *Male :* December 16th, 1850, 1 a.m., Birmingham (myopia, squints). *Male :* August 12th, 1849, 7.30 a.m.————(myopia). Dozens of similar instances could be given. *Male :* August 13th, 1850, 5.4 a.m., London. This is the nativity of the poet Philip Bourke Marston.

Ascendt.	☉	☽	☿	♀	♂	♃
♌ 23°14′	♌ 20°2′	♏ 1°30′	♍ 2°35′	♎ 0°18′	♍ 23°32′	♍ 24°6′

♄	♅	♆
♈ 20°54′ ℞	♉ 0°20′ ℞	♓ 2°0′

At four years of age he developed incipient cataract supervening upon inflammation. His sight gradually grew worse and was ultimately lost. The Sun is rising in Leo and receives the mundane [not zodiacal] squares of Luna and Uranus and the mundane semi-square of Mars. The Moon is opposed by Uranus from Taurus and receives the par. dec. of Saturn.

STONE IN KIDNEY AND BLADDER.—Gravel and stone are the result of the crystallisation and deposition of solid substances of the urine, and are usually the result of Saturnine action. This is the reason why such as are subject to the condition are often of the melancholy type and affected with hypochondriasis. In Chapter II. the kidneys are found to be placed under Libra, but the pelvis of the kidney under Scorpio. It is in the pelvis that stone is formed.

(1) *Male :* April 21st, 1822, 7 p.m., Lat. 51°N., Long. 7m.W. Here we find the first degree of Scorpio on the ascendant, and Sun, Moon, Saturn and Jupiter in close conjunction on the cusp of the seventh. Both luminaries receive a semi-quartile from Venus, and the latter planet bears a similar aspect to Saturn. It is true no planets are located in Scorpio. The influence

seems to be entirely reflected from Taurus. This pair of signs is singularly reversive in action, as we have remarked before. The positions are thus:

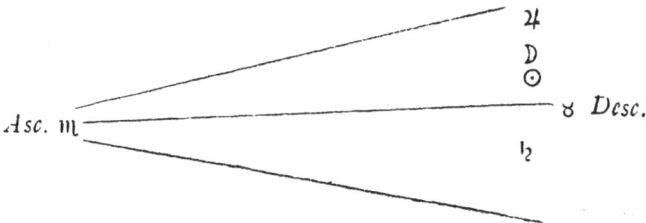

In this case stone in the kidney was only a secondary form of manifestation. The specific Taurian zone—the throat—was impressed with the greater evil—the resulting disorders being diphtheria, bulbar paralysis, and earlier in life quinsies and minor throat affections.

(2) *Female:* March 18th, 1852, 10.30 p.m., Lat. 52°30′N., Long 1°18′W. The figure shows ♏15° on the Eastern cusp, with a retrograde Jupiter rising in the same sign, but otherwise quite unafflicted. Venus, Saturn and Uranus are conjoined in Taurus and the sixth, and with this exception there is very little affliction in the horoscope. It would have been difficult to diagnose the complaint from the figure, but it is very significant considered by the light of the previous example.

(3) *Male:* November 7th, 1866, 4.30 p.m., Lat. 51°22′N., Long. 0°6′W. Stone in bladder. Stricture of urethra. Dyspepsia. Heart and back affected. Scorpio assumes its full dominion here. The last decanate of Taurus rises, and Sun, Moon and Saturn are conjoined in Scorpio near cusp of seventh. (They have passed the cusp and are nominally in sixth.) Venus is applying to a semi-quartile of Saturn. Mars is in Cancer on cusp of fourth. This latter accounts

for the stomach trouble. It is well to note that in kidney troubles Venus is usually associated with Saturn.

Asc. ♉ ————————————————————) ♏ *Desc.*
☽ |
♄ |
☉)

CHRONIC DIARRHŒA, CHRONIC INFLAMMATION OF BOWELS, ACUTE PHTHISIS.—*Male:* September 4th, 1864, midnight. Reference to the figure of birth will reveal abundant causes for the disorders specified. It will serve our purpose to present the main afflictions in the form of a diagrammatic tabulation in which they can be seen at a glance :

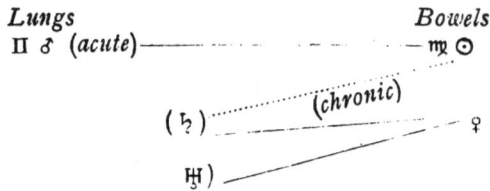

Lungs   *Bowels*
Ⅱ ♂ (*acute*)——— --- -- · -- · —♏ ☉
                       (chronic)
(♄) ············ —— ———— ——— -- ♀
♅) ——————

The connecting lines indicate evil aspects. The dotted line an evil aspect not quite completed. Planets in parentheses throw rays from other signs.

SCROTAL HERNIA, GRAVEL, DIARRHŒA, ANGINA PECTORIS, ACUTE NEURALGIC PAINS IN HEAD, KIDNEY TROUBLE AND BACKACHE.—*Male :* November 5th, 1855, 4.45 p.m., Lat. 52°28′N., Long. 7m.W. Uranus rises in Taurus, a very usual indication of darting pains in the head (origin obscure). Sun and Mercury are conjoined in the sixth house in Scorpio (*scrotum, bladder*), the former afflicted by a sesquiquadrate of Saturn, a semiquadrate of Moon (also in sixth), and an opposition of Uranus. Venus is in the sixth in Libra squared by Saturn. The scrotal hernia was due to the Uranian pressure ; the gravel to the Saturnian influence ; the angina to the predominance of fixed signs, and the occupancy by planets of fixed houses—Jupiter and Neptune eleventh, Mars fifth, Saturn second. The kidney trouble emanates from Venus in Libra squared by Saturn. Both luminaries are afflicted in the sixth house, and the native is a chronic sufferer.

CHRONIC BRONCHITIS, EPITHELIOMA OF NOSE (operation).—*Male :* June 21st, 1826, 1.5 a.m., Lat. and Long. as before.

Ascendt.	☉	☽	☿	♀	♂	♃
♉ 5°0′	♊ 29°3′	♑ 13°51′	♊ 24°33′	♋ 25°28′	♏ 5°17′	♍ 8°3′

♄	♅	♆
♊ 26°0′	♑ 23°2′	♑ 12°58′
℞	℞	

For the bronchial trouble we have heavy affliction in Gemini, the lung sign, intensified in action by the occupancy of the third house (equivalent to the zodiacal third). The type of disease is indicated by Saturn, *viz.*, chronic. For the epithelioma (the ultimate cause of death), we find Mars located in Scorpio (nose) exactly opposing ascendant, angular and consequently of great power. The perverted action of Moon in Capricorn (conjoined Uranus and Neptune), a sign connected with the epithelial tissues, should likewise be remarked.

CHRONIC BRONCHITIS, TUMOROUS GROWTH IN HEAD.— *Male :* May 25th, 1846, 0.5 p.m., Lat. 53°N., Long. 10*m*.W. For the bronchitis the Sun and Moon are conjoined in Gemini and receive the quartile aspect from Saturn in Pisces. For the tumour we observe Venus with Uranus in Aries squared by Mars from Cancer.

GASTRITIS, REMOVAL OF TONSILS. — *Female :* October 23rd, 1866, 0.40 p.m., Lat. 52°28′N., Long. 7*m*.W.

Ascendt. ☉ ☽ ☿ ♀ ♂ ♃
♏5°14′ ♎29°52′ ♈23°15′ ♏12°57′ ♐14°17′ ♋21°38′ ♑24°25′

♄ ♅ ♆
♏13°14′ ♋8°24′ ♈10°59′
℞ ℞

Mars angular in seventh; kinetic action to Sun in Scorpio (just leaving Libra); a fixed sign ruling the throat by reflection from Taurus. Great irritability of stomach. Gastritis. Martial and Uranian activity in Cancer.

BRIGHT'S DISEASE.—Acute and chronic desquamative nephritis will be usually accompanied by the ill association of Venus and Saturn. But as these maladies are not really due to some one form of morbid renal condition, the horoscopical positions may not show regular static energy in Libra. Sufficient cases have not come under the author's notice to enable him to draw satisfactory conclusions. But this much may be tentatively advanced: (1) Venus badly aspected by Saturn, (2) Venus badly aspected by Jupiter, (3) Sun badly aspected by Jupiter, (4) Moon occupying Cancer, Scorpio or Pisces, (5) Fixed signs prominent, but especially Scorpio, Aquarius and Leo, (6) Fixed sign rising. The reason for this prominence of fixed signs and the evil condition of Venus and Jupiter is not difficult to comprehend.

(1) Acute Bright's disease (complications). *Female :* April 17th, 1878, 12.35 p.m., Eye, Suffolk. The vinculi are seen to be as below :

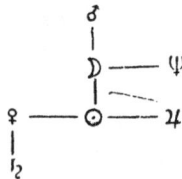

A fixed sign (♌ with ♅) rises. The Moon occupies a fixed sign (♏). Five bodies and the ascendant are located in fixed signs.

(2) Bright's disease, pneumonia, dyspepsia. *Male :* August 9th, 1836, noon.———— The pneumonia is primarily indicated by Mars in Gemini. The dyspepsia by Moon and Venus (afflicted by Saturn) in Cancer. For the albuminuria we have this planetary relationship : Venus and Jupiter in quartile with Saturn ; Jupiter opposition Neptune ; Moon in Cancer ; fixed signs prominent, *i.e.*, five bodies located in them and a fixed sign (♏) ascending. Saturn is just above the cusp. Approximate ascendant 3°♏ (owing to the latitude of birth not being available the exact degree cannot be determined).

(3) *Female :* January 4th, 1884, 1.15 p.m.———— The scheme shows Venus opposition Jupiter, par. dec. Saturn, Mercury and Mars, and applying to the opposition of the latter planet. Mars, Jupiter, Saturn, Uranus and Neptune are retrograde. The Sun is receiving the quincunx of Saturn and applying to that of Mars and finally Jupiter. The Moon is afflicted in Pisces. Fixed signs are well tenanted, five bodies holding possession. A fixed sign (Taurus) rises and Saturn is close to the cusp.

(4) *Male :* October 25th, 1833, 7.45 a.m., Lat. 44°50′N., Long. 0°34′W.

Ascendt.	☉	☽	☿	♀	♂	♃
♏20°	♏1°40′	♓24°12′	♏14°34′	♍29°57′	♏4°1′	♉0°24′ R

♄	♅	♆
♎4°57′	♒18°39′ R	♑26°43′

This instance exhibits Sun opposition Jupiter ; Moon opposition Venus ; Venus conjoined with Saturn (in the actual renal sign) and receiving a quincunx from

Jupiter. The latter body is on the cusp of sixth, retrograde, and afflicted by Saturn and Mars. Five planets occupy fixed signs, and a fixed sign is rising. The Moon is in Pisces. This case is also one of diphtheria, scarlet fever and cirrhosis of kidney. For the former see under the remarks on that disease, and compare the state of affairs with the examples there introduced. The principal consideration is that section of the figure here shown :

Cusp of Twelfth House.

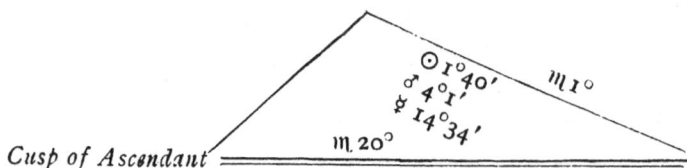

Cusp of Ascendant

MENTAL DERANGEMENT, EXAGGERATED EGO, ETC. —The mental rulers, Moon and Mercury, will both be afflicted, and usually in affliction with each other too. There are, however, many forms of mental trouble. Violent lunatics will be the outcome when Mars is the causative agent ; hypochondriacs when Saturn. There is also a class the subjects of which for a great part of their lives may exhibit brilliancy akin to genius in some direction, more particularly of the mechanically mathematical order, or where rapid calculation and mental subtlety are requisite. The primary responsibility rests upon the association of Mars with Mercury, especially by the conjunction and opposition. Many lightning calculators, chess players, inventors, mechanical geniuses, cranks, etc., have this position, the planets at the same time being located in one of the angles, or the third or ninth house. George Bidder, the celebrated calculating boy may be instanced (June 14th, 1806, 3.45 a.m.). Mars has just left the Moon (in Taurus) and is making appulse to Mercury; but in this case Saturn is in conjunction with Uranus, and the Sun in trine to both, while Venus, in Taurus, is in trine to Jupiter in Capricorn: Taurus is a sign peculiarly associated with mathematical ability. Gerard de Nerval, the poet and miscellaneous writer, had Mars conjoined with Mercury, but also opposed by Saturn. He committed suicide in a fit of insanity. Morphy, the chess player, had Mercury squared by Mars and Uranus. Rethel, the German fresco-painter, had Moon opposition Mars, Mercury opposition Uranus. George III. had Moon conjoined with Uranus and both squared by Mars. Mercury was also in conjunction with Saturn.

VARICOSE VEINS OF LOWER LIMBS.—These will frequently occur with Venus or Moon (or both) in Aquarius more or less afflicted, especially if there is Martial activity.

(1) *Female:* midnight, December 31st, 1864, Lat. 52°28'N., Long. 7m. W. Moon and Venus occupy Aquarius. The former is in close par. dec. with Saturn and applying to the quartile of Mars. Venus receives the semi-quartile of Neptune.

(2) *Female:* February 21st, 1826, about 10 a.m., same Lat. and Long. Venus and Mercury are in Aquarius on the cusp of eleventh (a house synchronising with the sign Aquarius). They are opposed by the Moon. Mars throws a cross quartile ray.

PULMONARY CONSUMPTION.—One or both luminaries occupy a common sign and a cadent house, particularly sixth or twelfth. There is general affliction in common signs and houses. Saturn and Mars evilly aspect luminaries according to type. In some cases Aquarius holds afflicted bodies, especially in acquired consumption and congestion of lungs.

(1) *Male :* March 15th, 1863, 7.45 p.m., Lat. 55°52'N., Long. 4°18'W. The Sun is in Pisces and on the cusp of sixth, a very frequent position with the consumptive. It is in par. dec. with and applying to the opposition of Saturn, in quartile with Uranus, quincunx with Jupiter, and almost in conjunction with Neptune. Mars and Uranus occupy the chief lung sign —Gemini. Saturn has passed into the twelfth house. When the latter planet completed its par. dec. with the radical Sun, and the Sun met the semi-quartile of the radical Mars, the native died (in his 26th year).

(2) *Male :* March 12th, 1864, 8.30 a.m., Lat. 52°40'N., Long. 1°20'W. The Sun again occupies Pisces, but this time on the cusp of the twelfth. It is also in par. dec. with Saturn as before, in quartile to Uranus in Gemini, and applying to the conjunction of Neptune. The throat, too, was affected. The moon is in Taurus and the twelfth, receiving the bad aspects of Neptune, Venus, Jupiter and Saturn.

(3) *Male :* December 6th, 1859, 9 a.m.———In this case the Sun is on the cusp of twelfth in Sagittarius. It is opposed by Uranus from Gemini, applies to a quartile of Neptune in Pisces, and receives in addition the semi-quartile of Mars. The Moon is in Aries much depressed by a par. dec. of Saturn, and having the opposition of Mars and the quartile of Jupiter.

(4) *Male :* August 16th, 1850, 1.30 a.m., Lat. 53°30'N., Long. 10m.W. Here it is the lesser light which is posited in a common sign (*Sagittarius*) and on the cusp of sixth. It bears the sesquiquadrate of Saturn and quartiles of Neptune and Mercury. The Sun is located on the cusp of third in Leo, Mars is conjoined with Jupiter in Virgo. Five bodies tenant common signs.

(5) *Female*: January 21st, 1855, 3 p.m., Lat. 54°40′N., Long. 5m. W. Pneumonia, from catching cold. Resolution being delayed, some degeneration in lung tissue took place and there were tubercular foci scattered through the lungs. Many complications. Heart failure and dropsy towards end. The Moon is conjoined with Neptune in Pisces and squared by Saturn in Gemini from cusp of twelfth house. The Sun is in Aquarius and par. dec. with Saturn. Five bodies in Aquarius.

A REMARKABLE CASE.

A most interesting study is afforded by the following geniture. The loose slip containing the figure fell out of an old copy of Lilly some years ago. There were no indications of time or place of birth, but these were evidently at 8.40 a.m. on October 4th, 1834, in or near London, the planetary positions being as below :

Ascendt.	☉	☽	☿	♀	♂	♃
♏6°45′	♎10°40′	♏0°42′	♎22°53′	♏27°5′	♋7°57′	♊11°41′ ℞

♄	♅	♆
♎13°0′	♒22°5′	♑28°50′

Scarlet fever, 1852 (Autumn). Gastric fever, 1859. Brain fever, 1866 (May). Fever, 1873 (July). Arm broken, 1869 (February). Severe blow or fall, 1860 (December). Cut thumb nearly off at seven years of age. Cut nose nearly off, 1862 (March).

G

CHAPTER XIV.

INDICATIONS OF SHORT LIFE.

THE indications of very early death are usually of easy remark to the astrologer. On the average the number of cases is small wherein such indications are liable to be overlooked or misunderstood, but these exceptions demand greater knowledge than we now possess.

It will naturally be expected that infants should suffer more from the severity of planetary influence than adults; that is to say morbid distemperatures will more easily result from evil transits, positions and directions, on account of the greater tenderness of the several parts. The period of life is indeed always to be considered in judging the effect of the stars as they form their various aspects by motion subsequent to birth. Old age, senility, have something like a parallel epoch in infancy, but the stellar effects are then of a different order, since the animal body by the actions inseparable from life undergoes a continual change: the smaller fibres become rigid, the minute vessels grow into solid fibres no longer pervious to fluids; everywhere there is a tendency to contraction, dryness and immobility, the true Saturnine principles.

Whenever the Sun is afflicted by Saturn, the vitality is low, and although one such testimony does not warrant the prediction of premature death, yet there is danger in the early years. It is important to remark the closeness of the aspect formed and whether *applicatio*

or *defluxus* is being made.   If the aspect is close, and
forming, the danger is accentuated.   In those cases, too,
where by what is termed " progression " or " direction,"
to be explained later, a planetary body will cross the
cusp of one of the angular houses (particularly the first or
seventh) in the early period of life, and where moreover
the vitality, as gathered from the Sun and Moon, is low,
a further testimony is provided.

Even where this transiting body is the Sun, Moon or
Jupiter, the disturbance produced is frequently such as
to bring disaster to the infantile organism.   And where
a malefic like Saturn is exactly on the oriental or
occidental cusp, or upper or lower meridian, a child is
often born dead or lives to inspire but a few lungfuls.

We must also bear in mind that some signs bestow
weaker constitutions than others, and persons born when
they are rising or are occupied by the Sun, have lower
vitality and prove more susceptible to the morbid effects
of planetary action, than those making their appearance
under signs of naturally strong constitution.   The weak
signs are Cancer, Capricorn, Pisces ; and in a general
way the whole of the common signs are less robust than
the fixed.

Again, a most critical epoch is the New Moon, and
before the contact is made.   To this lunar *bajamar* or
menguante much infantile mortality is referable.   The
weakness of constitution engendered by the position
renders any contemporaneous malefic conformation more
stringent still in its action upon the body.

The first case I take from the *Astrologers' Magazine
and Philosophical Miscellany* for October, 1793.   It is
there given to show the presumed importance of the *pars
fortunæ* as hyleg.   Hannah Parnel, March 11th, 1793,
12 p.m., " at a Mr. Matthew's, No. 16, Church Lane,
White Chapel."

Ascendt.   ☉   ☽   ☿   ♀   ♂   ♃
♏28°1′   ♓21°55′   ♓18°29′   ♓22°35′   ♉7°51′   ♈6°47′   ♐1°54′

               ♄   ♅   ♆
        ♈29°58′   (♌20½°℞)   (♏2½°)

" I calculated this nativity," says the writer, "when the child was about three weeks old, and informed the people of the house that it would scarce live half a year, though very different thoughts were at that time entertained by the child's relations. However, it did not live three months, but died on the first of June."* The Moon wants a trifle over three degrees to complete its conjunction with the Sun. Sun, Moon and Mercury are conjoined in a weak sign. Jupiter and Mercury are quite near to the cusps of first and fourth houses respectively. The Sun is in close par. dec. with Mars and semi-quartile Venus. Thus there are disclosed three of the testimonies previously enunciated as prospicients of early death, *viz.:* 1. Moon applying to conjunction Sun. 2. Sun (also Moon and Mercury) in a sign of semi-vitality (♓) and afflicted. 3. Bodies very near angle cusps.

A somewhat similar instance is afforded by the positions in the figure below. They are given from the chart which accompanied the communication, as neither latitude nor longitude is stated. *Female :* January 16th, 1828, 10.40 p.m. Died August, 1828.

Ascendt.   ☉   ☽   ☿   ♀   ♂   ♃
♎5°23′   ♑25°52′   ♑25°12′   ♑14°53′   ♒20°28′   ♏17°20′   ♏11°12′

              ♄   ♅   ♆
       ♋16°5′   ♑27°50′   ♑16°13′

1. The Moon is applying to conjunction Sun, being only 0°40′ of arc from completion. 2. The Sun afflicted

---

* The approximate positions of ♅ and ♆ have been added here although they did not of course enter into the writer's calculations.

in a sign of low vitality (♑): six bodies in signs of low vitality. 3. Bodies near angle cusps: Saturn culminating.

The next case shows a terrible array of evil aspects and positions. *Male:* December 21st, 1870, 7 p.m., Lat. 39°57′N., Long. 75°9′W.

Ascendt.	☉	☽	☿	♀	♂	♃
♌ 1°0′	♑ 0°0′	♐ 22°51′	♑ 15°51′	♑ 3°17′	♍ 26°41′	♊ 20°15′

♄	♅	♆
♑ 0°48′	♋ 25°36′ ℞	♈ 19°3′ ℞

Premature birth—six weeks in advance. Spinal meningitis, died January 1st, 1872. 1. Moon applying to conjunction Sun. 2. Sun afflicted in a sign of low vitality (♑): three other bodies in same sign too. 3. Neptune culminating and near cusp. 4. Note the heavy affliction of luminaries, quite sufficient in itself to negative the idea of life:

☉ ☌ ♄, ☽, ☿; □ ♂.—☽ ☌ ♄, □ ♂, ☍ ♃ ⊼ ♅

Female: March 7th, 1894, 2 p.m., near Canterbury. Died Autumn of same year.

Ascendt.	☉	☽	☿	♀	♂	♃
♌ 8°	♓ 17°1′	♓ 16°52′	♓ 28°41′ ℞	♒ 19°56′ ℞	♑ 15°19′	♉ 25°32′

♄	♅	♆
♎ 24°16′ ℞	♏ 15°13′	♊ 10°51′

1. Moon applying conjunction Sun. 2. Sun and Moon afflicted by par. dec. Suturn, quartile Neptune; Sun, Moon and Mercury are conjoined in a sign of low vitality (♓). 3. Saturn near cusp of fourth.

Occasionally the Press assists us. The death of a child after a life of twelve hours' duration necessitated the York coroner holding an inquest in March, 1903, at

Starbeck.　The little one was Christopher Turner, son of John Turner, goods porter, at Starbeck, Harrogate. The child was born on the 28th of March, at 1 p.m., and died on the 29th, from asphyxia, due to premature birth.

Ascendt.	☉	☽	☿	♀	♂	♃
♌ 12°50'	♈ 6°40'	♈ 0°34'	♓ 21°55'	♉ 4°55'	♎ 7°44' ℞	♓ 8°33'

♄	♅	♆
♒ 7°13'	♐ 25°38'	♋ 0°59'

The luminaries are heavily oppressed by Mars, Neptune, and Saturn.　In addition Uranus and Neptune throw quartile rays to the Moon, and Saturn is opposing the ascendant (in ♒—asphyxia), having just set.　Probably, the time of birth was a little earlier, when that body was exactly on the occident cusp.　The Moon is applying to the conjunction of Sun.

Male : October 12th, 1890, 9.32 a.m., Lat. 52°28'N. Long. 7m.W.　Died suddenly, January, 1891.　Occasioned a coroner's inquest.

Ascendt.	☉	☽	☿	♀	♂	♃
♏ 22°9'	♎ 19°0'	♎ 1°0'	♎ 1°27'	♐ 4°3'	♑ 12°19'	♒ 2°39'

♄	♅	♆
♍ 12°28'	♎ 26°34'	♊ 6°32' ℞

1.　The Moon applies to conjunction Sun, although more distant from that luminary than in the former map.　2.　The Sun is afflicted by Mars, Uranus and Venus.　3.　Saturn is transiting the mid-heaven.

ARCS OF DIRECTION.

Where planetary bodies are close to one of the angle cusps the arc of direction to that cusp is important, operating powerfully upon the child, and, when tokens of short life obtain, usually indicating the exact time of death.

For instance, in the above figure the Arc of Direction* required is a little over 0°14', since the rate of measurement is 1°=1 year, or 15'=3 months.   To determine this we say :—*Right Ascension* Saturn 164°28'27", less the *Right Ascension of the Mid-Heaven*164°14'0",equals Arc of Direction " M.C. ♂ ♄ , *in Mundo* "—0°14'27".

Another direction operative at the time was Moon conjunction Mercury, *d.d. zod.*   The conjunction falls in 1°27' Libra, *Dec.* 0°34', with a *R.A.* of 181°19' and a *Semi-arc* of 89°17'.

Moon's Semi-arc	95°22'	Prop. log.	(*arith. comp.*)	9·72419
Moon's Meridian Distance	18°39'	,,		·98810
Semi-arc Aspect	89°17'	,,		·30450
Moon's Second Distance	17°19'	,,		1·01679
M.D. Aspect	17° 5'			

ARC OF DIRECTION   0°14' Moon conj. Mercury, *d.d. zod.*

Another example.   *Female :* September 1st, 1894, 9.18 a.m., Latitude and Longitude as before.

Ascendt.	☉	☽	☿	♀	♂	♃
♎ 20°40'	♍ 8°53'	♍ 29°57'	♍ 7°5'	♌ 15°58'	♉ 3°35'	♋ 2°6'

	♄	♅	♆		
	♎ 22°21'	♏ 12°5'	♊ 15°44'		

The affliction obtaining here, as regards the three centres—Sun, Moon and Ascendant—we find to be Sun conjunction Mercury (afflicted by Saturn, hence malefic),

---

* For a full explanation of the meaning and use of these and other terms relative to this part of the subject the reader is referred to Part IV. of *The Progressed Horoscope*.   Manual V. of this series gives, however, a very clear outline of the principles involved, with illustrations of the methods employed.

semi-quartile Saturn, quartile Neptune. The Moon has just left the Sun, is in quartile with Jupiter and semi-quartile Venus. Saturn is on the the cusp of ascendant. The child died on the 29th of October, 1895, of consumption. Note the affliction in lung signs. If we now compute the arc of Saturn to conjunction of ascendant we shall have the time of *terminus vitæ*. The *R.A.* of Saturn is 201°31′, the *Semi-nocturnal Arc* 99°31′, the *M.D.* 98°22′. Then *Semi-arc* of Saturn 99°31′ minus *M.D.* Saturn 98°22′ equals 1°9′, the Arc of Direction "Ascendant conjunction Saturn *in mundo*." This, at the rate of one degree per year, and five minutes (*of arc*) per month, reaches exactly to the time when the event transpired.

Male : July 26th, 1895, 9.45 a.m., Lat. and Long. as before.

Ascendt.	☉	☽	☿	♀	♂	♃
♎0°13′	♌3°7′	♎1°6′	♋13°41′	♏17°39′	♌28°18′	♋21°31′

	♄	♅	♆
	♏0°57′	♏15°51′	♊17°15′

The above figure exhibits the Sun afflicted by semi-quartiles of Neptune and Venus, and a quartile of Saturn. The Moon is on the first house cusp, semi-squared by Uranus. From the latter position one would expect something peculiar in connection with the head. As a matter of fact there was a curious malformation of the skull : a longitudinal depression in central part and on either side soft, watery, hemispherical excrescences. This child died, April 1896, of bronchitis complicated with measles.

Male : March 15th, 1898, 3.50 p.m., Lat. and Long. as before. Consumptive, died November 18th, 1899. Notice that no fewer than six planets occupy lung signs and that the luminaries mutually afflict each other, the Sun itself being posited in the "house of death."

Ascendt.	☉	☽	☿	♀	♂	♃ .
♍ 2°30'	♓ 26°6'	♐ 29°29'	♓ 24°9'	♈ 1°57'	♒ 25°40'	♎ 6°43'

	♄	♅	♆
	♐ 12°15'	♐ 3°31' ℞	♊ 19°48'

The Time Factor.

Planetary Periods, Climacteric Years, etc.

It is well to note that there are certain fairly well-marked planetary periods governing the life. Thus, from birth to the fourth year is dominated by the Moon; the 4th to 10th by Mercury; the 10th to 18th by Venus; the 18th to 37th by Sun; the 37th to 52nd by Mars; the 52nd to 64th by Jupiter; and onwards from the latter year, by Saturn. The deductions from this are pretty obvious. Evil, directions of the Moon during the lunar period will be especially dangerous; those of Mars in the Martial period; those of Saturn in the Saturnian; and so with others.

Not only this, but there are the climacteric years to be observed, for such epochs are undeniably disastrous to organic equilibrium. They are especially to be considered when malefic directional aspects are in force. The accompanying diagram will exhibit the planetary life-periods and the lunar critical epochs (p. 106).

In this diagram the "three score years and ten" of the psalmist are represented as the arc of a semi-circle, the radial lines indicating the time of expiry of the influence of one planet and the commencement of the one which succeeds it.

The ten chords divide the arc into seven-year sections, which have a double significance in relation to the life. Firstly, the Planet Uranus completes his cycle in eighty-

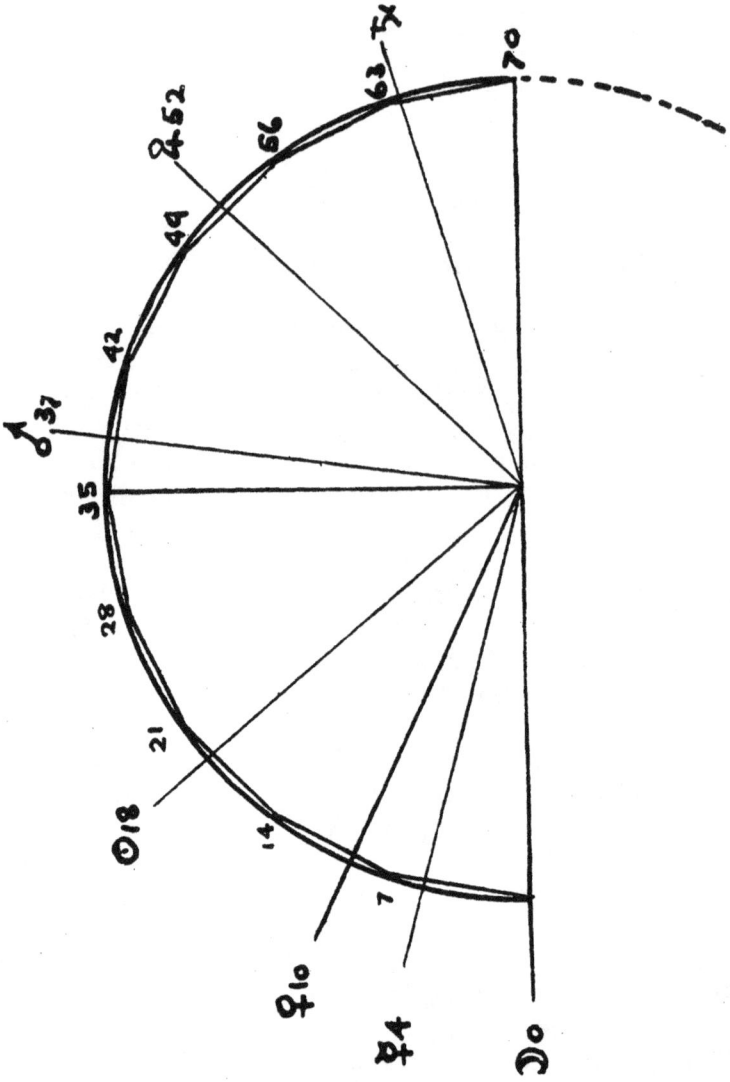

THE PLANETARY AND CLIMACTERIC PERIODS.

four years, or one sign in seven years, and thus takes up a position ⅴ, ✳, ▢, △, etc., his radical place, every seventh year after birth.   Secondly, and this is perhaps of more importance in direct relation to health, the effect of the progress of the planets after birth is felt by means of what is termed the " progressed horoscope," in which the movement of the planets each *day* after birth is found to affect the corresponding *year* of life.   Since, then, the Lunar Quarters so important in the animal economy occur each seventh day or thereabouts, we can thus easily see how the life will be mapped out into *seven-year* periods of correspondingly greater importance in. the life of man.

And here it seems pertinent to mention that every lunar month typifies the circle—birth to death, generation to fruition and decay.   There is consequently a monthly renewal and dispersion of force, *bios*.   It is only in the more fluent forms of matter that the influence is pronouncedly apparent, nevertheless all grades of matter are affected.   There is a tide of the bodily fluids as well as of the ocean, a period of activity and repose, a systole and diastole, times of preparation, development, perfection and disintegration.   All these are represented by the lunar phases.

The NEW MOON implies disintegration, death, preparation for a new cycle.   It is the low ebb, the *nitya pralaya*, the systole.

The *First Quarter* is concerned with organic development and the revitalisation of function and fluid.

The FULL MOON typifies fruition, maturation, high tension, fluidic plenitude.   This is the lunar expiration and diastole

The *Last Quarter* is devoted to the application of power already generated.   The reaping of the harvest.

The medullary and cerebral substance is augmented

at the full, and suffers diminution at the new. The size and weight of the brain depend very much upon the relation between the luminaries at birth, being smaller at the new and increasing to the maximum at the full. Likewise on account of the plenitude induced at the latter epoch, many plethoric and other effusions and emissions are brought about, *viz.*, catamenia, hæmorrhoidal and allied sanguineous discharges and evacuations, epistaxis, hæmorrhage, hæmoptysis, malæna, etc.

In certain febrile disorders which run their course in a short time, there occur critical days. These depend upon the lunar aspects formed with the place of the Moon when the illness seizes one. This latter time is known as the " decumbiture " among the older astrologers. The aspects in question are the semi-quartile, quartile, sesquiquartile and opposition, and of these the principal are the quartile and opposition, formed about every seventh day. The temperature and pulse of the patient frequently obey closely the sway of these periods.

[The Second Manual of this Series, *What is a Horoscope and How is it Cast?*, gives clear elementary information concerning the Casting of a Horoscope, and also hints as to its judgment when cast. Fuller information will be found in *Casting the Horoscope* and in *How to Judge a Nativity*.

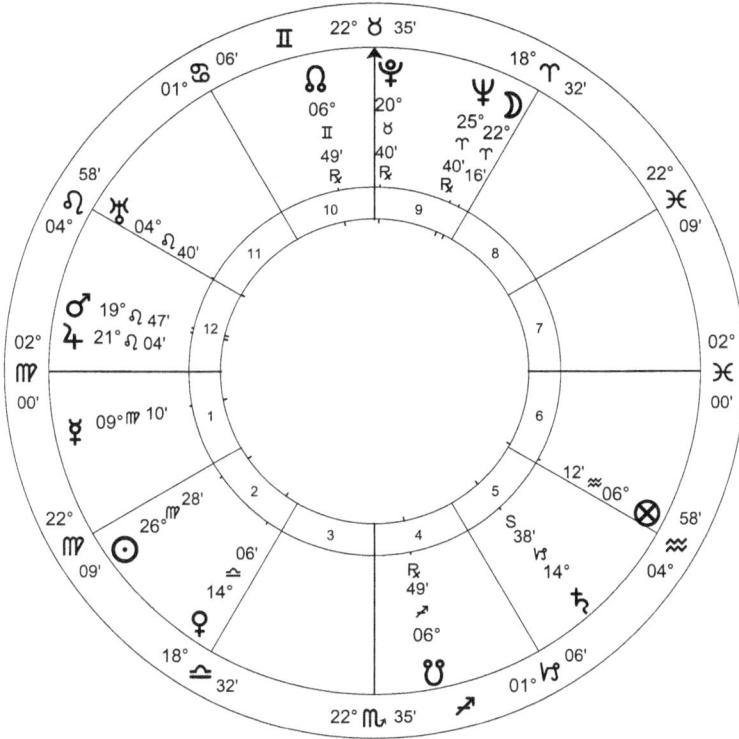

Natal chart of Heinrich Däath
Born September 19, 1872
3:28 am GMT
Peterborough, England.

Other books on Medical Astrology and related subjects, published by Astrology Classics / AstroAmerica.com

David Anrias: **Man and the Zodiac,** *1938*

E.H. Bailey: **The Prenatal Epoch,** *1916*

*Joseph Blagrave***: Astrological Practice of Physick,** *1671*

Luke Broughton: **The Elements of Astrology,** *1898*

C.E.O. Carter:
The Astrology of Accidents, *1932*
An Encyclopaedia of Psychological Astrology, *1954*

H.L. Cornell: **Encyclopaedia of Medical Astrology,** *1933*

Nicholas Culpeper: **Astrological Judgement of Diseases from the
    Decumbiture of the Sick,** *1655, and,* **Urinalia,** *1658*

William Lilly: **Christian Astrology,** books 1 and 2, *1647*
    The Introduction to Astrology, Resolution of all manner of questions.

Richard Saunders: **The Astrological Judgement and Practice of Physick,**
    1677

upcoming:
Dr. M. Duz: **A Practical Treatise of Astral Medicine and Theraputics,** *1912*

Better books make better astrologers.
Here are some of our other titles:

AstroAmerica's Daily Ephemeris, 2010-2020
AstroAmerica's Daily Ephemeris, 2000-2020
 - *both for Midnight. Compiled and formatted by David R. Roell*

Al Biruni: **The Book of Instructions in the Elements of the Art of Astrology**, *1029 AD, translated by R. Ramsay Wright*

David Anrias: **Man and the Zodiac**

Derek Appleby: **Horary Astrology: The Art of Astrological Divination**

E.H. Bailey: **The Prenatal Epoch**

Joseph Blagrave: **Astrological Practice of Physick**

Luke Broughton: **The Elements of Astrology, 1898**

C.E.O. Carter:
The Astrology of Accidents
An Encyclopaedia of Psychological Astrology
Essays on the Foundations of Astrology
The Principles of Astrology, *Intermediate no. 1*
Some Principles of Horoscopic Delineation, *Intermediate no. 2*
Symbolic Directions in Modern Astrology
The Zodiac and the Soul

Charubel and Sepharial: **Degrees of the Zodiac Symbolized**, *1898*

H.L. Cornell: **Encyclopaedia of Medical Astrology**

Nicholas Culpeper: **Astrological Judgement of Diseases from the Decumbiture of the Sick**, *1655, and,* **Urinalia**, *1658*

Dorotheus of Sidon: **Carmen Astrologicum**, *c. 50 AD, translated by David Pingree*

Nicholas deVore: **Encyclopedia of Astrology**

Firmicus Maternus: **Ancient Astrology Theory and Practice: Matheseos Libri VIII**, *c. 350 AD, translated by Jean Rhys Bram*

Margaret Hone: **The Modern Text-Book of Astrology**

Alan Leo:
The Progressed Horoscope, *1905*
The Key to Your Own Nativity, *1910*
Dictionary of Astrology, *edited by Vivian Robson, 1929*

William Lilly
Christian Astrology, *books 1 and 2, 1647*
 The Introduction to Astrology, Resolution of all manner of questions.

Christian Astrology, book 3, *1647*
Easie and plaine method teaching how to judge upon nativities.

George J. McCormack: **A Text-Book of Long Range Weather Forecasting**
With Foreword by David R. Roell, Astrology At Our Feet

Jean-Baptiste Morin: **The Cabal of the Twelve Houses Astrological**
translated by George Wharton, edited by D.R. Roell

Claudius Ptolemy: **Tetrabiblos**, *c. 140 AD, translated by J.M. Ashmand*

Vivian Robson:
Astrology and Sex
Electional Astrology
Fixed Stars and Constellations in Astrology
A Beginner's Guide to Practical Astrology
A Student's Text-Book of Astrology, *Vivian Robson Memorial Edition*

*Diana Roche***: The Sabian Symbols, A Screen of Prophecy**

*David Roell***:**
Skeet Shooting for Astrologers
Duels At Dawn, the second book of essays
Triple Witching Hour, the third book of essays
Quad Bike Analysis, the fourth book

Richard Saunders: **The Astrological Judgement and Practice of
   Physick**, *1677*

Sepharial:
The Manual of Astrology, the Standard Work
Primary Directions, a definitive study
Sepharial On Money. *In one volume, complete texts:*
   • **Law of Values**
   • **Silver Key**
   • **Arcana, or Stock and Share Key** — *first time in print!*

Zane Stein: **Essence and Application, A View from Chiron**

James Wilson, Esq.: **Dictionary of Astrology**

H.S. Green, Raphael and C.E.O. Carter
Mundane Astrology: *3 Books, complete in one volume.*

————————————————————————————

If not available from your local bookseller, order directly from:
The Astrology Center of America
207 Victory Lane
Bel Air, MD 21014

on the web at:
http://www.astroamerica.com